eat.de

Advance Praise

'It's a mother's wish to have someone who cares – and I can assure you Pooja does.'

– Genelia Deshmukh

'*Eat Delete Junior* is designed so that children don't bite off more than they can chew.'

– Mandira Bedi

'*Eat Delete Junior* helps you help your kids make better choices.'

– Shaheen Abbas

eat.delete.
junior

Child Nutrition for Zero to Fifteen Years

POOJA MAKHIJA

with
Gayatri Pahlajani

HarperCollins *Publishers* India

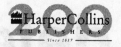

First published in India in 2017 by
HarperCollins *Publishers* India

Copyright © Pooja Makhija 2017

P-ISBN: 978-93-5264-487-2
E-ISBN: 978-93-5264-488-9

2 4 6 8 10 9 7 5 3 1

Pooja Makhija asserts the moral right
to be identified as the author of this work.

The views and opinions expressed in this book
are the author's own and the facts are as reported by her,
and the publishers are not in any way liable for the same.

It is recommended that parents check with their child's paediatrician
before following the advice in this book.

HarperCollins *Publishers*
A-75, Sector 57, Noida, Uttar Pradesh 201301, India
1 London Bridge Street, London, SE1 9GF, United Kingdom
Hazelton Lanes, 55 Avenue Road, Suite 2900, Toronto, Ontario M5R 3L2
and 1995 Markham Road, Scarborough, Ontario M1B 5M8, Canada
25 Ryde Road, Pymble, Sydney, NSW 2073, Australia
195 Broadway, New York, NY 10007, USA

Typeset in 11/14 Baskerville
by Jojy Philip, New Delhi

Printed and bound at
Thomson Press (India) Ltd

To Badi and Chotti,
For giving birth to another me

Contents

Alice in Wonderland

I woke up in an unfamiliar room. It was dark. A tree branch was scratching against the window. What I thought was the moon was in fact a fluorescent streetlight, angling in through the grill, the ghostly light making a pattern on the wall, one that looked a bit like a tablecloth. A head seemed to emerge from behind the tablecloth, asking me if I was feeling better. Was the tablecloth speaking to me? And feeling better from what? I went back to sleep.

When I woke up again, it was daylight. The room was now

devoid of tablecloths – both speaking and non-speaking – to be replaced instead by a reassuringly human non-table-clothy man who looked suspiciously like my ob/gyn. 'Hey,' I said, 'you look a lot like my doctor.' To this he replied, 'That's good, because I am your doctor.' And then it hit me, the reason for the disorientation, the pain, the discomfort and the strange room with my doctor in it – I was in a hospital and I'd just given birth. And if that were true, where was the fruit of my labour? My eyes started darting around looking for their apple.

'My baby?' I croaked.

My husband suddenly emerged from behind the curtains around my bed like the final act of a hastily penned murder mystery. To further amplify the drama, he dragged a screechy cot with him. But, as it turned out, it was only the chariot for my beautiful baby girl. Ah, my baby girl: ten wiggly fingers, ten wiggly toes. Bundle intact, I began to cry because that is what you do when your husband pops out from behind the curtains with your firstborn. Sensing her mother's senility going south, my daughter then began to cry. Or it could have been time for a feed.

Despite the pretty-in-pink pictures and tonnes of text available on the subject, nothing in the world that you have read, watched or been counselled on will ever prepare you for having a child. Whether you've given birth, had a surrogate or adopted a baby, you – and only you – will be able to understand exactly what you felt when you first set eyes on your child. You can go to Mars, win a Nobel Prize, find the cure for the common cold, but nothing will ever come close to that moment when you're holding your baby in your arms for the first time. It is also that moment when you realize that your life has changed and will never be the same again. Having a child is like a fairy tale. Where you're Alice in Wonderland. And where becoming a parent is your rabbit hole.

The reality of parenting starts to hit you as soon as the painkillers wear off. It is overwhelming. Your life had order and structure; now it won't. You had time for yourself; now you don't. Nothing will make sense for a while. A full night's sleep becomes a distant memory and going to the bathroom becomes a decision that you need to plan, strategize and think over. Nothing will prepare you for the sheer quantum of advice lobbed in your direction either. The only way I can describe it is to compare it with walking on the road on your way to an appointment when suddenly a vehicle going past splashes dirty ditchwater all over your hair, your face and, of course, your outfit. Which is white.

I'm not comparing advice to ditchwater, although that is what it may seem like at first. Some advice is brilliant and has saved me – and my kids – time and again. Here I refer more to the unexpected timing of it, which can really feel like a slap on the face. A blissful mummy-and-baby moment on a plane, for example, can be hijacked by someone in your row who will list the benefits of Benadryl for travelling babies and, not-so-subtly, for other passengers too. Or when you're at the supermarket and Junior wants you to put her up on the cart and have you push her down the sabzi aisle going 'wheeeee', someone will comment on whether that's really good for your child. Doctors' waiting rooms, fitting rooms, women's loos and the odd funeral, no place being free of unsolicited 'feedback'. You get advice from the help at home, shopkeepers and drivers too. And, sometimes, even from those who have never had a child.

New parents are not always the best recipients of this deluge of advice. As a first-time mother, for example, how do you look for answers when you don't even know what the questions are? You're grappling with your very new baby, a very new surge of hormones, a very new feeling of exhaustion and sleep deprivation, all coupled with the feeling that you are not doing it right, even though you are. Parenting can also make you feel judged. You feel the world's eyes on you because you're the only source of nutrition, values and security for your kid for a long time to come. Things said lightly as a joke – visitors commenting on how the baby looks absolutely nothing like you or, worse, how you still look pregnant after giving birth (I've experienced this one) – can make you feel sensitive. You feel vulnerable and insecure. You are trying to do your best, and even the most well-meaning advice can make you feel like you are being scolded.

You are not alone. According to a recent study conducted in India[1] a massive 90 per cent of Indian mothers feel that they were under pressure to be the perfect parent.[2] Based on my personal experiences and interactions with my clients, I'd say that figure is way off base. I'd peg it closer to 100.

Given the circumstances, one more book telling you what to do then may seem counterintuitive. But that is not why I wrote this. I wrote this because new parents are bombarded with confusing and, sometimes, misleading information. It is becoming difficult to reach a consensus because what sets each of us parents apart is our children's unique bio-individuality, even as what unites us is our intention to always do the best for them. To that end, I'd like to use this book as a way to clarify not confuse, to prioritize not pressurize, to reassure not rile, so that things become clearer and anxiety levels go lower. The problem with overwhelming access to information online is it can be precisely that: overwhelming. And even though the truth is that nothing is more fundamental than nutrition – it is literally what propels your child's development, his brain function, his motor skills, pretty much his entire existence – *Eat Delete Junior* has been designed to calm parents down by separating the bogus from the beautiful, so that you learn exactly what needs to be done and what needs to be left alone.

This book will also expand on eating behaviours because *what to eat* is only one aspect of nutrition – *how to eat* is another. If your child is a picky eater, for example, making life a living yell at dinnertime, are you to sit back while your kid puts very little or no food in her mouth? It is hard to be Buddha-like about a situation where your child's nutrition is compromised, sometimes even dangerously. Or what about older children and their uncanny superpower-like ability to search and latch on to junk food? Malnourishment can happen even if your child is eating all the time. As a parent, it is important to know how to deal with it.

So keep calm and read. Or, at the very least, keep calm. Being a nutritionist and a mother, I can happily tell you that, unless specified, everything in *Eat Delete Junior* has been tried and tested either on my own two girls or on my little clients. I can also tell you that there is absolutely *no* nutritional problem without a solution and there is no child who won't eventually respond. The advice here has been designed to appeal to those parents who already know a lot about child nutrition – through their environment or copious after 2 a.m. red-eyed online readings of the subject – and for those who don't know as much. No matter which level of knowledge you're coming in at, this book will help clarify and crystallize your thought process, put some myths to bed, surprise you with something you probably didn't know and simplify your approach to feeding your child until, of course, he or she can feed themselves and make nutritionally responsible decisions.

There are thirty-four children born in India every minute.[3] That's 2062 births per hour and about 49,481 per day. And each one of them is a question mark. A bawling, cooing question mark. You really don't know what you're getting. Or, if you're a first-time parent, what you're getting into. You've given birth to or adopted the biggest question mark of your life – what kind of person will they be? Will they sleep through the night? Will they be a demanding toddler? Will they know how to take care of themselves? Will they be a well-adjusted adult?

While we may not be able to answer all of life's questions, *Eat Delete Junior* has been designed to address child nutrition in India like few other books have, because it is customized to both Indian foods and cultural contexts. It is compact, it is simple and it will be your go-to guide for everything nutritional, so that mealtimes become that time when your child gets the best. Both out of food and out of you.

How to Use This Book
Blitz through Your Read of *Eat Delete Junior*

Honestly, I would recommend reading the whole thing from start to finish, but for those who want to just skim through because they are strapped for time and patience, look out for these signs:

> **Mini contents pages:** For those of you who only want to read what is relevant, I've provided a tool to turn to the appropriate page. To that end, I've sub-divided the chapters into mini contents pages with page numbers, which will be within a box, like this one. Look out for the dashed box.

The megaphone indicates a very important point, so look out for this sign. I originally wanted to choose a gossipy old aunty to represent this element – since I needed to symbolize something really good at broadcasting information – but after serious thought, I went with the megaphone instead.

This represents the summary of each chapter, the ABCs as it were. The synopsis may overlap with the megaphoned information but if you don't have time to read anything else, dip into this section at least.

There are also mini chapters inserted between the main chapters that are designed in reverse, i.e., white text on a black background, so do look out for them. Their purpose is to highlight a point that is, at least according to me, too significant to be quietly tucked away in a chapter, and you'd do well to read these.

Other notes on *Eat Delete Junior*

I have tried to make the book gender neutral, so at any point parents of a boy or a girl would be able to relate to that information. I have done that by making the child a 'he' in one chapter, and a 'she' in the next, so that both genders have equitable representation, just like I feel they should in real life. It is a small point but I wanted to bring it out in my book.

I have been working in nutrition for over fifteen years and been a parent for about twelve of them, and I can tell you before you start reading *Eat Delete Junior* that it is best if you don't aim for perfection. You may read something and realize that you have been doing it differently all this while. You may attempt some techniques and then figure out that your child just isn't responding as quickly as you would like him or her to be. The information you find in the pages of this book has been designed to make your and your child's life easier; so do keep that in mind. Also, the book has been demarcated by age, but it doesn't always mean that the advice is strictly meant for that age group alone. It doesn't matter whether you are breastfeeding or if your child is already a tall, strapping teenager, you will find something of value in this book. Enjoy the read and, most importantly, enjoy the journey.

Breastfeeding

It is a unique privilege. As a new mother, you are essentially your newborn's supermarket, ice cream, comfort food, cheat day, artisanal snack, canapé and those precious mini cupcakes with the little hearts on top. In other words, you are his nutritional universe. When you are breastfeeding, you are your child's only means of satiating his hunger, quenching his thirst and fulfilling – to a large extent – his primal need for security. Breastfeeding is one of the fastest ways to start feeling like you are a mother and it is a position of both awesome power and pretty much awesome responsibility. Which is why you don't want to get it wrong. Which is why you are driving yourself crazy.

Don't.

I prescribe lactation diets for new mothers so they can nurture themselves and their newborns at the same time. But while it all sounds good in theory, I am usually confronted with something that looks a bit like this:[1]

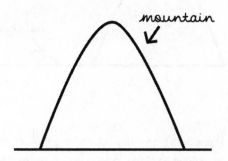

No, I haven't lost the plot entirely. At least not today. The picture above is of a mountain, as the arrow very helpfully suggests. New mums come in with their foreheads almost constantly creased during their appointments with me, bringing with them mountains of concern, doubt and unwarranted fear. Sometimes they bring with them people having mountains of their own: mothers, mothers-in-law or sisters, who are all equally worried. While I would strongly advise you not to call any of them a mountain, I would also like to point out that I am not dismissing the concerns of first-time mothers, because I was one myself. And no matter how old your children are, it is hard not to recall the stress, the uncertainty and the worry about one of the most primal and nurturing functions of human existence: breastfeeding. What I am trying to say is that you don't *need* to. If the main area of concern is about how to produce a steady stream of milk for your newest consumer, I can tell you right now that your nutritional concerns usually need to look a bit like this:

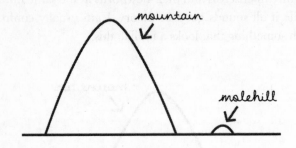

mountain

molehill

There aren't too many nutritional guidelines at the breastfeeding stage and it is best to appreciate this phase of your life for what it is: a magical time.

Breastfeeding is a unique opportunity to bond with your baby, something that you will never share with your child again. This is the stage where you firmly establish the stubborn belief that no man/woman will ever be good enough for your daughter/son and your baby is probably the best one that ever lived. It is also a period of cracked nipples, immense sleep deprivation, snapping at the husband and trying very hard not to snap at the mother-in-law. It can be wonderful, exhausting, special, magical. And it is over all too soon.

From a dietary perspective, don't confuse yourself with too many dos and don'ts, wrongs and rights. Yes, it is better if you take good nutritional care of yourself but you don't have to obsess over this phase and drive yourself to the point of despair. You already have a lot on your plate. Just keep in mind, though, that as breastfeeding is the first nutritional decision you make for your child, **understanding the role of your own nutrition** in making milk is the best starting point to this beautiful phase of your life.

But first, let's understand what we are dealing with. When you give birth, a surge of hormones – namely prolactin and oxytocin – at the time of delivery will lead to the production of breast milk. This is irrespective of whether the baby has come into the world via C-section or through vaginal delivery. The act of separating the placenta from the uterus causes a hormonal shift, which in turn sends a message to the mammary glands[2] to produce milk. In other words, you are ready to feed almost the second after you give birth to your baby.

Ideally, while it is best to put the baby to breast within the first hour of delivery – clearly no wasting time here – it has been found that mums who have had stressful or traumatic births have a tendency to not be able to produce milk so quickly[3] because the anxiety inhibits their 'let-down' reflex. However, wait longer than an hour post delivery and it is possible that babies will find it harder to latch on and the possibility of nipple engorgement could be higher. Either way, if it is hard to breastfeed within the first hour, your doctor would probably advise you to pump and feed as soon as you are able to.

Breast milk is nutrient-rich and is pretty much all an infant needs for the first six months of his life for growth and

Feeling Let Down by Your Let-Down?

The let-down reflex makes the milk in your breasts available to your baby. This reflex is caused by a chain reaction: the baby's sucking at the breast triggers nerves which, in turn, trigger the hormones prolactin and oxytocin that cause the breast to 'let down' the milk. Sometimes, the let-down reflex can simply be caused by seeing, hearing or thinking about your baby. In addition to this, touching the breast and nipple area or using a breast pump could also trigger the reflex.

What the let-down reflex feels like:

1. A tingling sensation that can be strong
2. Fullness of the breast
3. Milk dribbling from the other breast
4. Contraction of the uterus, especially if you are not a first-time mother
5. Change in the sucking pattern of the baby from quick sucks to a more rhythmic suck-and-swallow movement

While the let-down reflex usually takes place more than once in a feed in response to the suckling of the baby, most mothers don't always notice it after that first time. The let-down feeling sometimes goes away after the initial few days or weeks.

It is said that your let-down may not work well in moments of anxiety, pain and exhaustion, or if you are upset. So, if your let-down reflex has let you down, try to:

Unwind. Take a deep breath, both literally and figuratively. Use other techniques which could help you relax, like a warm drink (milk or something non-alcoholic), music or a few rounds of pranayama if you are so inclined. A warm shower or bath or warm water on the breast just before you start feeding could work. A shoulder or back massage might also help with the relaxation. Whatever works for you.

Massage. You could also stimulate the reflex by massaging your breasts towards the nipple with a flat hand or a finger's edge. You could also try to slowly roll the nipple between your fingers.

Think. Since the reflex also depends on how you feel and is not just physiological, spend a bit of time thinking about your baby, **especially** while expressing. Visual stimulation, like an image of your baby, can also help. Look at a picture of him if he is not physically present, and just at him while he is.

Source: https://www.breastfeeding.asn.au/bf-info/early-days/let-down-reflex; last accessed on 16 February 2017

development. When you are breastfeeding your baby, you are giving him:[4]

1. Free water
2. Protein, which includes urea, peptides, nucleotides, free amino acids and DNA
3. Fats, which include fatty acids and long-chain PUFA (polyunsaturated fatty acids)
4. Carbohydrates, essentially lactose
5. Minerals, trace elements and vitamins

In short, you are giving him everything a little human needs for growth and development.

Breast milk is also packed with antibodies, antimicrobial factors and enzymes for digestion, growth factors and hormones,[5] and is a brilliantly unique food that cannot be replicated. And it is adaptive too: if your child is sick, antibodies in the milk automatically adjust to meet the baby's requirements.

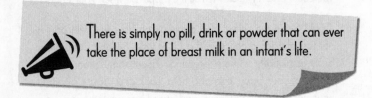

There is simply no pill, drink or powder that can ever take the place of breast milk in an infant's life.

There are three individual stages of lactation. They are as follows:[6]

1. **Colostrum:** Less milk, more secretion, colostrum is what is produced in the first seven days post the delivery. It has a high amount of protein, not as much fat, and contains vital immunizing components for the little one.
2. **Transitional Milk:** It is when the actual production of milk in the breast tissue occurs and is a graduation from the colostrum stage. This usually starts from Day 8 and goes on till Day 20.
3. **Mature Milk:** This is the real-deal breast milk. It starts from Day 20 onwards, and has about 65-70 calories per 100 ml. The fat received by the infant gradually increases as the feed continues. The mature milk continues the good work of providing immunity factors and other important elements to the baby.

For ease of assimilation, I have broken up this chapter into two parts. The first part, **Eating for Feeding**, will talk about what you can eat through this phase of your child's nutrition. The second part, **Feeding**, will talk about your baby and his relation to the nutrition he gets.

Part One

Eating for Feeding

I. The Role of Nutrition in Breast Milk

If you are a stickler for definitions like I am or, at the very least, would like to upstage your fellow breastfeeder with some extra information, do know that those foods or drugs which promote or better the flow of breast milk are called **galactagogues**. The nutritional galactagogues for milk are protein, water and sugar; the three are synthesized by your body to make breast milk.

Protein   Water   Sugar

$$= P + W + S$$

When considering what to eat, I would like to start off by saying that **you don't need to drink milk to make milk.** For those who think that the consumption of milk is in itself reassurance that breast milk is being produced, it is the protein, water and sugar present in the milk which is doing that, not the milk itself.

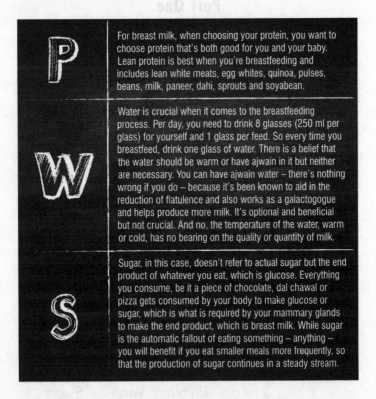

For breast milk, when choosing your protein, you want to choose protein that's both good for you and your baby. Lean protein is best when you're breastfeeding and includes lean white meats, egg whites, quinoa, pulses, beans, milk, paneer, dahi, sprouts and soyabean.

Water is crucial when it comes to the breastfeeding process. Per day, you need to drink 8 glasses (250 ml per glass) for yourself and 1 glass per feed. So every time you breastfeed, drink one glass of water. There is a belief that the water should be warm or have ajwain in it but neither are necessary. You can have ajwain water – there's nothing wrong if you do – because it's been known to aid in the reduction of flatulence and also works as a galactogogue and helps produce more milk. It's optional and beneficial but not crucial. And no, the temperature of the water, warm or cold, has no bearing on the quality or quantity of milk.

Sugar, in this case, doesn't refer to actual sugar but the end product of whatever you eat, which is glucose. Everything you consume, be it a piece of chocolate, dal chawal or pizza gets consumed by your body to make glucose or sugar, which is what is required by your mammary glands to make the end product, which is breast milk. While sugar is the automatic fallout of eating something – anything – you will benefit if you eat smaller meals more frequently, so that the production of sugar continues in a steady stream.

If the above seems like a head-scratcher, given that it is a bit broad, below is a sample meal plan for lactating mothers, modelled around the diets I prescribe to my new mothers in their first six weeks post delivery, where weight loss is not the focus. The focus here is more on recovering from the delivery process, including healing of stitches, returning the hormonal cycle to the pre-pregnancy state, contraction of the uterus, establishing good breast-milk production as well as basically coming to terms with your changing life. It is not a hard-and-fast rule but basically a recommendation. Like I said, there is no major nutritional tectonic shift you need to make; there will be only some calorie addition.

SAMPLE LACTATION PLAN

6 a.m.:
- 1-2 glasses of water
- Soaked almonds + walnuts or small laddoo (wheat or ragi) with some nuts (sweetened with dates or dried figs, not sugar)

8 a.m.:
- Vegetable juice (introduce this 2-3 weeks post delivery)
- Vegetable upma or poha (with sprouted fenugreek seeds) or cereal with milk/yogurt
- Or egg whites with bread or roti

10 a.m.:
- Oats/ragi/cracked wheat porridge sweetened with dates/fruit

12 noon:
- Masala chaas (fresh yogurt) with cumin powder and mint leaves
- Roti – wheat/bajra/jowar/ragi with cumin seeds or methi (fresh or seeds) (like a masala roti) and/or rice
- Vegetables – methi (fenugreek)/ bottle gourd/ drumstick veg/dill leaves (shepu)
- Dal – moong (initially and then gradually introduce all types) or fish or chicken

2 p.m.:
- Fruit + milk or chaas

4 p.m.:
- Herbal tea (tulsi/cumin/ajwain/methi/fennel seeds or saunf)
- Crackers or khakra

6 p.m.:
- Soup (vegetable or chicken) with toast/khakra

8 p.m.:
■ Similar to lunch

10 p.m.:
■ Milk with kesar and/or elachi with biscuit

12 midnight (if awake):
■ Fruit or crackers (with ajwain) or nuts (if not had earlier in the day)

When I prescribe lactation diets like the one above, I usually add on about 500-700 extra-nutritious, hardworking calories that help both mother and baby, but the number of calories depends on the mother. Breastfeeding women need to bump up both the quality of nutrients and the quantity of food to enable the synthesis of milk, even while the resultant calorie increase may be quite minimal for some women, which is why the above meal plan is just a general guide. The number of calories a mother needs depends on her level of body fat and how active she is.

In the absence of a nutritionist, the best way to customize these diets for yourself is to first calculate your Basal Metabolic Rate (BMR). Your BMR is the minimum number of calories your body needs for it to perform its most basic functions like breathing and sleeping (yes, these burn calories too). BMR calculators are available online but if you are more of a pencil-and-paper kind of person, you can use the Harris-Benedict equation. The one below is for women:

$$BMR = 655.1 + (9.563 \times \text{weight in kg}) + (1.850 \times \text{height in cm}) - (4.676 \times \text{age in years})$$

Alternatively, as the point of *Eat Delete Junior* is to simplify things for harried and busy parents, you could also just do a quick calculation on any good BMR calculator online. Once you have calculated your BMR, add about 500-700 calories to that and it becomes your daily nutritional need. If the 500-700 calorie spectrum seems a bit broad, then add 500 first and see how you are doing. The next step, of course, is to find meal plans which correspond to the calorie count that your BMR + extra calories has suggested. So, for example, if your BMR is 1500, adding 500 calories to it means you will need to look for a nutritious, healthy, 2000-calorie diet.

While you can also find these online or by asking your own nutritionist, I thought I would provide some sample diets that correspond to your calculated BMR + calorie addition. You will find these in the Appendix (page 199).[9] Do note that the extra calorie addition is not simply about adding empty calories but also giving nutrition to your baby and to yourself, which you will need as part of the healing and feeding process in the months to come. Also, the meal plans have been prescribed keeping in mind a breastfeeding mother's schedule from 8 a.m. to 2 a.m. and have taken into consideration what she has access to late at night as opposed to what she can prepare for herself – or have someone help her prepare – through the day.

But this is also the part where I highlight how sock-you-in-the-guts fabulous mother nature is. Even if you, as a mother, are struggling to manage good nutrition, nature will *always* protect your baby. But there is a catch: it will be at your cost. If a mother's diet is falling short for whatever reason – be it access to good nutrition, poverty or disguised malnutrition in which the mother is not eating right – her body will plug the gap by giving to the baby by *taking from her body.* If your baby isn't getting enough calcium, your body will leech it from your bones and give it to him. If your baby isn't getting enough protein, your body will tap into your muscles and give it to him. If your baby isn't getting enough carbohydrates, your body will exhaust your glycogen stores to compensate for the lack of carbs in the breast milk. That is how nature is – it will ensure the survival of your baby. It has been seen that even in the poorest of countries, in cases bordering on malnutrition, breast milk is still nutritionally adequate for the baby even if his mother is struggling for it.

But that is not reason enough to go wildly off-course, of course. Why would you want a situation where your health is being compromised? Where your calcium is being leeched or your muscles are being weakened, putting you within spitting distance of osteoporosis or muscle dystrophy? Or where reducing glycogen stores reduce your energy and take the joy out of your life? Why shouldn't you enjoy nursing as much as your baby does? What is the point of motherhood if you don't cherish it most of the time? Even if your health is not motivation enough to eat right – although it should be – you must, at the very least, take care of yourself because you are taking care of a tiny being too. If this chapter was a telegram, the message would read: 'Tiny Being Dependent on Giant

Eating for One

I hate to be the bearer of bad news but pregnancy-related cravings are a myth. The only truth that exists in this context are pregnancy-related *aversions*. Cravings are psychological but aversions are physiological. While you may have loved certain foods, you might just hate them as your pregnancy progresses. And vice-versa too. Your distaste for celery sticks could become a staple during your bun-in-the-oven days, so expect the unexpected. Also note that during pregnancy, your nutritional needs only marginally increase and that too every trimester. You do not eat for two. You eat for one.

Human'. You are the giant human, no disrespect. You are the first port of call for your baby, no matter how involved your better half is. Ergo, by default, not taking care of yourself is not taking care of your baby.

II. Quantity of Milk

Of the crease-deepeners that deepen the creases on most mother's foreheads, this one is the deepest. New mothers constantly worry about milk production, about 'drying out', about somehow depriving their baby of nutrition. The reality of it is that they needn't worry. When it comes to quantity, a mother doesn't need any particular food to bump up the supply of milk.

 Your baby's sucking will dictate how much milk needs to be produced. Your *baby* will decide the quantity.

But since I am on this page, I am hoping to get all my readers on the same page too. I wanted to use this space to break a few myths about milk supply in the form of questions that I get asked by my new mothers during their consults:

'Pooja, I'm not getting enough hindmilk. What should I do?'

You do nothing. Generations of women have nursed generations of scientists, geniuses, statesmen, leaders and the odd astronaut without knowing the composition of their breast milk; so it is best not to worry. The question is not without a valid basis, yes, but it all comes down to the same thing in the end. Let me explain: to start with, for those who aren't in the know, the nature of breast milk can change during the same feed. **Foremilk** is the initial phase of the feed. It has higher water content. **Hindmilk** is the latter part of the feed which has greater fat content. The fat received by the infant gradually increases as the feed continues. Needless to say, you want your little bundle of joy to receive more of the fatty, good stuff; so more hindmilk.

The imbalance between foremilk and hindmilk takes place when the breasts either have too much milk in them or if the feeds are strictly timed. To put it simply, the emptier the breast, the more fat content in the milk; the fuller the breast, the more the initial watery foremilk. This is why feeds that are later in the day have more fat content while those earlier in the day are more diluted. The reason I ask my clients not to worry about the quantum of fat in milk is that if you feed your baby on demand – whenever he asks for it – as opposed to timing it, the overall feeds for the day will give the baby the fat he needs. Which is why I also tell my clients that if they haven't heard of the foremilk-hindmilk concept to begin with, then they should best consider it unheard. Feed your baby whenever he wants and all will be well. It is important to note that **all breast milk has at least some fat**.

 If you haven't heard of the concept of foremilk-hindmilk, it is best to leave it that way. Your baby will get all the nutrients he needs in the end.

'Pooja, I'm expressing but I don't seem to produce enough milk. Does this mean that my baby is not getting enough?'

Nope. That is not true either. The fact of the matter is that you cannot measure how much milk you have. There are many who breastfeed beautifully but cannot express. A baby at the breast provides stimulus for the breast to push out the milk, the **let-down reflex** as mentioned earlier. In other words, the baby gets more when he is feeding directly – because he triggers the reflex – as opposed to when breast milk is expressed and given from the bottle.

'When's the best time to feed? Should I wait for my breasts to fill up with milk?'

There is no 'best time' to feed. Any time is mealtime for baby boo. Having said that, there is an advantage if you breastfeed at night. Prolactin, the hormone that sends the signal to the breasts to make milk, is the highest at night because it follows a circadian rhythm (a circadian rhythm has been defined as a twenty-four-hour cycle for physiological processes in all living beings including plants, animals and humans). So night feeds are good for milk supply. They also ensure that mother and baby have close contact round the clock, which helps in the baby's brain development. But even though night feeds are advantageous, do note that:

 There is always milk if your baby wants it because your breasts make milk all the time.

How fast your body makes milk, though, depends on how much your baby wants it. The more he wants, the more you will make.

'Do soft breasts mean no milk?'

It doesn't. The feeling of fullness/hardness in your breasts in the initial weeks post-delivery may disappear. Many of my clients worry that if their breasts feel soft or if they cannot feel the let-down reflex, it means their breasts don't have milk, but that is not true. In reality, your body is adjusting to your baby's needs and produces milk accordingly, so your breasts don't always have to be full.

The milk supply also depends on how balanced and nutritious your diet is. But if it isn't, there are over-the-counter galactagogues (preferably take those which are Ayurvedic or natural in preparation, like fenugreek powder), which may increase your milk supply. If you are eating a balanced diet, you don't need these. But if your doctor is okay with it, it is okay with me. Do note, though, that galactagogue powders have *lots* of sugar (possibly to kick-start milk production), which means that they are pretty high in calories and should be used judiciously. You could also incorporate some of the following galactogogue foods as ingredients or as part of the main dish:

List of galactagogue foods
1. Garlic
2. Fenugreek seeds and leaves
3. Sesame seeds
4. Coconut water (electrolyte plus hydratant)
5. Cumin seeds
6. Fennel seeds
7. Tulsi
8. Bottle and bitter gourd

9.   Drumsticks and its leaves
10. Poppy seeds or khas khas
11. Oats
12. Dill leaves (shepu)
13. Salmon or indian rawas
14. Edible gum or gondh
15. Water

III. Vitamins, Minerals and Supplements

In a balanced, nutritious diet, your baby is getting his daily dose of vitamins and minerals from what you are feeding him, so it is usually not a cause for concern. For example, breast milk contains a small dose of iron that is easy for babies to digest.

But my issue is mainly with two major vitamins which are not too abundantly available. If you are on an especially vegetarian diet, consider taking Vitamin B12 supplements, but only on the say-so of your doctor. B12 is found exclusively in animal products – which includes meat and dairy – and is hard to find in vegetarian diets. Don't forget to account for this, though, because B12 is incredibly crucial for the brain development of your infant.

It is also very likely that you would need Vitamin D because most of us have low levels of it. Just you yourself don't need this vital vitamin, your baby does too, as it helps absorb calcium and phosphorus, which makes his bones strong. A lack of Vitamin D, as we know, can cause rickets – a disease that softens or weakens bones (although it is more common in severely malnourished children). Vitamin D supplements can also be given to babies, but for this you need to have your paediatrician in the know.

Whatever you choose, do not self-medicate where supplements are concerned because despite their warm and fuzzy image, an overdose of supplements could cause toxicity, especially if they are fat soluble like Vitamins A, D, E and K.

IV. Foods to Avoid

There are no foods to avoid while breastfeeding. Not even one. Traditional wisdom flies in the face of this, though: while breastfeeding, the mother should make sure there is no besan, no beans and no anything-that-passes-gas-onto-the-baby in her diet. But nutritionally, the rule of thumb is that if *you* cannot digest it, your baby won't. If you cannot tolerate beans and legumes – and you get gassy – don't expect your baby to as well. If you can digest food that is thought to be indigestible or gassy by many, good for you. And for your baby. You don't need to keep scrutinizing your diet. Babies don't always have gas because of something you ate. What you could digest one day may not be that easy to digest on another. You may not have eaten differently, but your baby may react to it.

Thirty-one-year-old Sameera had just given birth a week before when her baby started screaming post a feed. It turned out he was gassy, poor thing. She had inadvertently eaten some besan kadhi prior to that and attributed his crying to what she ate. She came to my clinic still haunted by the experience, worried about making another misstep. Don't be. Be kind to yourself. The key is to treat the entire nutritional phase of breastfeeding as trial-and-error. Don't be terrified or wracked with guilt if you have made your baby gassy or kick-started a marathon of tears (not just yours). If you are a first-time mother, you are as new to this as he is. Accidents are accidents and I can speak from experience when I say that guilt will not make you a better parent. A constructive and happy outlook will.

And no, you don't have to keep your ears covered to make

non-gassy milk (there is a theory that air coming into the ears – like Superman – will somehow make breast milk gassy). Keep your ears covered, though, if you want to drown out the sound of your crying baby from time to time. Or to drown out the advice of one more person telling you to cover your ears.

V. Alcohol, Smoking and Lactation

While science is still figuring out whether drinking while feeding leads to drunk babies, they can't walk in a straight line anyway so I figure you will never really know. Bad jokes apart, what some studies have suggested is that alcohol in the breast milk impacts the baby's ability to drink properly, which in turn impacts their growth.[7] That alcohol is a galactagogue happens to be a bit of an old wives' tale, I'm afraid, and it doesn't do much for your let-down reflex.

Just like it enters the bloodstream, alcohol quickly enters breast milk as well. If you are exclusively breastfeeding, it is best not to drink until your feeds are at least four to six hours apart, and even then try to stick to a 90-ml glass of wine. Chase this with two glasses of water to flush out the alcohol from your system and wait at least four to six hours before you embark on the next feed. I would avoid sugary cocktails entirely if I were you because they are heavily calorific and usually use higher-proof alcohol, which takes longer to leave the body.

But doing the maths is all too complicated. A simpler way to deal with alcohol while breastfeeding is to bypass the breast entirely if you decide to drink. Plan your next drink by expressing pure, 'non-alcoholic' breast milk *before* you raise that glass and feed the baby through a bottle later, so you have a greater gap between the alcohol entering and leaving your body.

No smoking while you are breastfeeding, I'm afraid.

HOW MUCH SHOULD YOU WEIGH?

Losing the Baby Weight

There is a feeling among some new mothers – like myself at the time – that during labour, the bulging stomach will move from the 'first floor' to the 'ground floor' and somehow delivery will 'concave' nine months of 'convex', resulting in a flat stomach. I hate to be the bearer of bad news but that simply doesn't happen.

During pregnancy, a part of the weight gained is evolution's way of providing an 'energy deposit' so that your body can cope with the demands of breastfeeding. So some of the extra post-pregnancy weight will hang on like an uninvited guest because your body needs it. However, the good news is that the process of synthesizing milk increases your metabolic rate, which burns calories as you continue to breastfeed. Many of the extra pounds will gradually be used up during the course of breastfeeding, so you should lose some weight during that time as well, assuming you are managing your diet well. Breastfeeding also releases oxytocin, which will help the uterus contract and lead to further loss of inches on your 'abs'.

For the kilos and inches that you can't shake off during breastfeeding, do wait at least six weeks post an uncomplicated delivery before you make a dedicated effort for weight loss. Your body needs time to recover from the trauma of delivery as well as to get into the rhythm of making good milk (for hormones to come back to pre-pregnancy state so that weight loss can start). Lose weight slowly while you are breastfeeding because you need to have adequate nutrients to feed your child along with the energy to take care of him. Lose no more than a pound or kilo a week with a balanced nutritious diet and exercise.

Part Two
Feeding

I. Feeding on Demand

I still remember the precision with which my eldest fed. She used to feed on the dot every two hours during the initial months of her birth. Not 1.55 or 2.05, but exactly every two hours. I used to put her down to sleep after a feed, only to be woken up precisely two hours later; I made a game out of counting down the minutes. I seriously wondered whether this clockwork feeding was the result of her listening to me tell my clients to eat every two hours − about thirty times a day, six days a week − for about nine months. She must have received the message in utero and was probably trying to make me happy after springing out into this world. How sweet. But then, daughter #2 came along and did nothing of the kind; her feedings were not at all timed. Well, so much for my theory, brilliant though I thought it was.

But it is best to understand more about why newborns seem to be eating all the time. Let's assume that the black blob below is your newborn bundle of joy's stomach. Ergo:

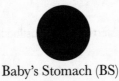

Baby's Stomach (BS)

Of course, it won't make sense at all unless you put it in scale.

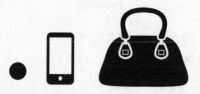

From (L) to (R) Baby's stomach, cellphone, handbag

While investigations are underway to understand how that particularly gruesome image of the handbag got into this book, the point, of course, is to make a point. That your baby's stomach is incredibly tiny. The tinier it is, more frequent the feeds and lesser the amount of time you will spend between them. So it is important to feed when he asks for it. And when I say 'asks', I mean bawl. He is hungry.

But you know all this and you wonder why I am telling it to you. The simple point is that babies are born with their own survival instincts, their own needs and their own limits for satiety. And these very newborns evolve into toddlers, then little children, then teenagers and finally adults with their own survival instincts, their own needs and their own limits for satiety.

But I would like to use this opportunity to state a point so important that I wouldn't mind if the book was titled that instead: **obesity starts at the breastfeeding stage.** Let me say it out loud one more time with the help of my trusty megaphone.

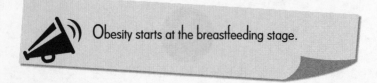

Obesity starts at the breastfeeding stage.

What I am trying to say – for the third time apparently – is that feeding practices in infanthood can dictate feeding practices in adulthood, leading to developing habits where the adult ignores satiety signals or that feeling of being full because it is what he did during his childhood. And ignoring satiety signals is not something that can easily be corrected. It is best to feed babies when they specifically ask for it, when you have figured out the difference between your baby's hunger cry, boredom cry, diaper cry and the I'm-so-lonely-pick-me-up cry. Forcing a baby to eat, even at the breastfeeding stage, could lead them to override their own feelings of fullness. As you may already know, signs that your baby is full during breastfeeding include physical detachment, lack of interest in the breast as well as unclenching of the fists, which now look looser and more relaxed.

The main issue here, of course, is to address the perception that a chubby baby is a healthy baby. It is not always the case and could, in fact, be a marker for an unhealthy one. I will tell you what I mean: our bodies have fat cells. Yes, we curse them and all, but we do need them. Fat is needed for insulation, the regulation of body temperature, protection of organs, among other things. About 60 per cent of our brain is fat.[8] The growth in fat tissues – or adipose – is what leads to adding more love to your love handles as well as to other areas of fat distribution. So we need them, yes, but we don't need them that much.

Adipose increases because of two reasons: the number of fat cells (hyperplasia) and the size of the fat cells (hypertrophy). These cells are used to store lipids (fats) and greater the amount of fat stored in a cell, the larger its size. Obesity therefore occurs when either the number of fat cells increase (hyperplastic obesity) or when the size of the fat cells grow (hypertrophic obesity) or even both. In this way, fat has two ways to deposit itself in the body, quantitatively and qualitatively.

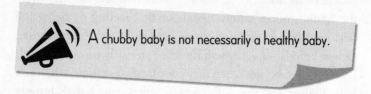

A chubby baby is not necessarily a healthy baby.

From birth, the size and number of fat cells grow in the baby, tripling or quadrupling until he reaches the age of two. In non-obese children, the size and number of fat cells remain more or less stable till another spurt in the number during puberty. However, in obese children, after the age of two, there is an additional increase in the number of fat cells, leading to what is sometimes called – especially in our culture – puppy fat. It is not always the case that puppy fat is shaken off as the child gets older because while it was once believed that the number of fat cells did not increase in adulthood – thereby helping a child to 'grow' into his height – new evidence[9] shows that it can.

Why fat cells grow in size and number can be attributed to a specific reason in some cases. For example, a rare reason would be a tumour located in the hypothalamus, which could prompt overeating. But in most cases, this growth can either be linked to genes – over which we have no control – or to one crucial reason over which we do have control: our eating habits. The way we eat, or overeat, could influence the number and size of fat cells, and it has nothing to do with how we are born.

In fact, it could all boil down to one's environment. Research suggests that adoptive parents who are obese can raise an obese child, irrespective of the gene pool.[10] In other words, if the environment around the child promotes overeating, that child is more likely to do so, developing a potential to be obese in the future. This could be due to the fact that if we eat excess fat, it gets stored in our fat cells. But if we eat more fat than our fat cells can accommodate, new ones can be formed to store that fat. Once formed, the number of fat cells remain the same, no matter how much we diet or exercise. They may only reduce in size.[11]

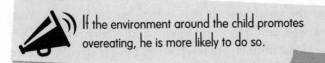

If the environment around the child promotes overeating, he is more likely to do so.

Simply put, how we eat contributes both to the number and the size of fat cells. And how we eat starts as early as breastfeeding.

Studies suggest[12] that something as innocuous as feeding through a bottle could result in a baby eating more than he needs. While bottle feeding has been designed to mimic breastfeeding with the shape of the nipple and so forth, it is actually not the same thing. The baby has to work less when he is feeding through a bottle because the milk flows more readily than with the breast. This is also why, as adults or older children, it is important to chew your food well, so the brain gets the signal that you have had enough. Effort = satiety.

The baby's role becomes more passive when being fed with a bottle and, as a result, the chances of overfeeding are higher. In bottle feeding, control also moves from the baby to the mother, thereby reducing the baby's ability to regulate how much he actually wants and needs. Limited evidence also suggests that bottle-fed infants gain weight far quicker than breastfed infants, enhancing their risk for childhood obesity. Yikes!

Bottles are still needed, though; it is just not practical to not have them. They are a crucial part of a mother's bag of tricks and a vital lifesaver for an exhausted parent. But the thought I am trying to convey is that bottles need to be used with vigilance. Signs of a baby reaching satiety levels need to be recognized even during bottle feeds, irrespective of whether the bottle has formula or expressed breast milk.

But the good news is that babies *can* self-regulate. Your baby knows how important food is and is born with his very own survival instinct. He has his own hunger signals, his own feedback, his own comfort zone and he knows what is needed. Stuffing your baby just to reassure yourself that he is 'fed' has more to do with *your* assessment of your baby's hunger levels than his. We feel the need to ensure the child is full based on *our* parameters – the emptiness of a bowl or bottle – but not the child's parameters, the feeling of fullness in his stomach.

For me, this is such a crucial point that I will now mark the start of every chapter with the proportionate size of the baby's stomach, so that you have a constant reminder of how important this is.

Because your baby's body has been designed to accept only so much.

II. Formula

I have yet to meet a mother who didn't want to breastfeed her child, but it is not always easy or practical to do so. Ambitions to solely breastfeed can sometimes violently clash with basic human responses like tiredness and lethargy. In some cases, access to breast milk becomes difficult, or even impossible, especially if your baby is adopted or via a surrogate and to

that end, in some cases, formula may be your only choice.
Having said that, many people prefer formula and top feeds so
while your paediatrician will be the best judge on how much
to give your baby, I thought I would include some formula-
feeding guidelines. The following are **daily allowances**, so
do distribute them between feeds:

In the first week:
> 60 ml per kilo per day, no more than 30 ml per feed

From the second week:
> 150 ml per kilo per day, no more than 60 ml per feed

At the age of one month:
> 150 ml per kilo per day, no more than 90–120 ml per
> feed

The above will continue from the age of one month to
one year. Formula will continue at 150 ml per kilo per day.

As an alternative or as an adjunct to any formula-feeding
plans, I would express breast milk and freeze it, creating my
own little bank of it. When I needed to draw on my bank, the
container was taken out of the freezer – it can be stored for
weeks or months on end – thawed and brought back to room
temperature. **Breast milk should never be heated.**

Creating a Breast-Milk Bank[13]

I thought I would lay out the dos and don'ts of making your
very own breast-milk bank in the Appendix (page 197). A stock
of frozen expressed breast milk can be stored for up to a *year*.
Making a breast-milk bank could also help free you up to let
other people feed your baby in your absence and is especially
useful for mothers getting back to work. Needless to say, baby
feeding at the breast is best for self-regulating the feed, but
expressed breast milk works beautifully as an adjunct.

Mix Up Bottle and Breast

If you think of introducing the bottle, do it early, else there will be too much dependence on the breast. But overdependence on the bottle could lead to your baby rejecting the breast. In short, mix it up.

Types of Formula[14]

It bothers me that the plural of baby formula is unfortunately not 'baby formulae', and many a minute was spent frantically searching this online. While one shouldn't cry over spilt minutes or formula for that matter, I still think the right option looks wrong. But let's move on. Not all types of formula are created the same way, and include many options that work for different times in a baby's life. I have included a few below, but please check the usage with your paediatrician.

Zero to Six Months: Grade 1 Formula

Grade 1 formula is composed of 60 per cent whey and 40 per cent casein. Examples of brands found in India include NAN Pro 1, Similac Advance 1, Enfamil 1 and Lactodex 1.

Six to Ten Months: Grade 2 Formula

Grade 2 formula has a 50 per cent whey, 50 per cent casein ratio. Examples of brands include NAN Pro 2, Similac Advance 2, Enfamil 2 and Lactodex 2.

Ten Months to Two Years

At the ripe old age of ten months, your child may need to switch to formula that is fortified with iron, or with EPA and/or DHA, both of which are omega-3 fatty acids. The whey:casein ratio may stay the same.

I would also like to point out that the above does not

constitute an endorsement of any brands but is just based on my general research.

III. When to Stop

When breastfeeding your child, there really is no set-in-stone rule for how long you need to keep feeding. Whether you continue till your child is six months, twelve months or even older (the World Health Organization [WHO] believes that children can be breastfed till they are two years old), this is extremely specific to the mother and the child. And the doctor, of course, while we are at it. What I can do is tell you when I stopped and my reasons for doing so.

For me, ten months was the magical age when I decided my babies' nutritional needs were being amply met through solid foods and they were able to enjoy the process of nourishing themselves through non-breastfeeding means. From the time of introducing solids to my daughters at the age of six months till they reached the ten-month mark was a comfortable window to slowly replace breast milk with solids entirely. Through my experiences with my clients, I also find that many mothers postpone the weaning process because breastfeeding can sometimes be the easiest way to put the baby to sleep, as breastfeeding is not always about nutrition; sometimes babies just want to feel secure. To them I say, 'Do whatever works for you and your baby,' but the more disciplined you are in weaning your baby off breast milk, the better it is for you both.

Whenever you decide to stop, know that this is truly one of the most magical phases of your life, despite the difficulties that come along with it. Most mothers love the gratification of breastfeeding; there is just something about that bond and the nurturing and the love. It can be the biggest joy on earth because it puts you in the unique position of being both the creator and the nurturer. It is a heady and humbling feeling. I think women are very lucky to experience it: the cracked nipples and mind-numbing exhaustion excluded. However, not everyone feels the same way. It can be extremely difficult, physiologically taxing and even traumatic for some mothers, so it's a very personal decision for a very personal act.

Before we move on to the next chapter, Introduction to Solids, there is one last thought that I want to leave you with. According to a National Institutes of Health (NIH) study, the baby first 'tastes' food via amniotic fluid in utero: the dual senses of taste and smell are already functional in foetuses. Because the foetus swallows amniotic fluid from time to time, this means that it gets direct access to 'transmittable' flavours, influencing the acceptance of solid foods in the future.[15] The same study found that pregnant women who drank carrot juice for three weeks continuously in their last trimester gave birth to babies who made fewer negative facial expressions when first introduced to carrot-flavoured cereal over regular cereal, indicating easier acceptance. It has also been found that some flavours imbibed by the lactating mother appear in breast milk, like garlic, vanilla and alcohol. Therefore, what you eat could subtly change the flavour of the breast milk, and the baby starts to imbibe an understanding of flavour difference as he grows. Eating from a wide variety of food groups and cuisines exposes your baby to different tastes.

His diet is introduced first through the womb, then through breast milk and later through his environment. So if you want your kid to eat everything, you should too.

THE ABCs OF BREASTFEEDING

Chapter Summary

There are no great nutritional changes you need to make for the breastfeeding phase. But it is better if you eat healthy; eat lean protein and small meals more frequently.

You will never run out of breast milk. You will make it as long as your baby wants it. Having said that, nighttime feeds produce the most milk.

If you haven't heard of the foremilk-hindmilk concept, consider it unheard. All breast milk has at least some fat in it.

Both Vitamins B12 and D are not commonly present in food and vegetarians may especially have limited exposure to B12 in their diets. Supplements work well to make up for the shortfall of these vital nutrients. Check with your doctor before consuming them, though.

There are no foods that you need to avoid while breastfeeding, but if a particular food makes you gassy or cannot be digested by you, expect your baby to have the same reaction.

Alcohol has to be limited to one glass of a lower-proof drink like wine and there should be a four to six-hour gap between drinking and feeding. No smoking while breastfeeding, though.

Feed on demand, i.e., when your baby needs it. It is best not to assess your baby's needs using your own parameters – the emptiness of a bottle. Overfeeding at this most tender age could lead to obesity later as babies become children who learn to ignore their satiety signals.

 A chubby baby is not necessarily a healthy one.

 While the feeding of formula is a conversation you may need to have with your paediatrician since it does depend on your baby, do consider building a breast-milk bank to accompany or completely replace formula.

 While when to stop breastfeeding is a personal decision, I find that ten months worked well for my daughters.

 Your baby can taste flavours both in the womb and in breast milk, paving the way for easier acceptance – and less opposition – of various foods later. If you want your child to eat everything, you must too.

Once Upon a Time

How Your Relationship with Food Affects Your Children

I have it on good authority that all adults were children first. And once upon a much earlier time, we were often patiently reminded that if we didn't finish our meals, we were wasting food. Many times when we looked forlornly at an equally forlorn half-eaten chapatti staring back at us from our plate, we were gently told by the supervising adult that we were blessed to have food on the table. Meals in our house, for example, often started with a prayer thanking God for the food we were about to eat. In the stricter households of friends growing up, eagle eyes would be fixed on them lest they take flight mid-meal. Once upon a time, finishing all the food served was an integral part of disciplining children.

It is now another time. Or is it?

Your established relationship with food can potentially influence your child's relationship with it, especially if it is something you aren't aware of. If we were taught to clean our plates of food, we are more likely to instinctively do the same thing in turn as adults and pass on the torch, perpetuating the cycle. Of all the reasons to eat food, polishing your plate because that is how you were raised may be the most harmful one. This simple, innocuous rule may not only lead you to ignore your own satiety signals, but it may lead to your children ignoring theirs. Or you ignoring theirs if they protest.

Every human being has their own unique biodiversity and it is supremely important to understand it. Each person's level of fullness, activity and attitude towards food differs and while genes definitely have a role to play, so does the environment your child was raised in. As articulated in the chapter on breastfeeding, an environment that promotes overeating or forced feeding is more likely to produce an overweight or obese child. But I'm a realistic kinda gal and have reasonable expectations both from myself and others. I don't believe that behaviours, which have taken years to establish and been influenced and reinforced by cultural norms and customs, will change overnight.

 What I would just like to do here is simply promote an idea: it is important to *feed* mindfully and not just eat mindfully.

The next time you prepare food for your child or are about to embark on feeding one, try and spend a minute on how you were raised, your culture, your relationship towards food or even your own body image. For example, parents who were once overweight children can be paranoid about calorie intake in their own young ones since they don't want them to have experiences of being bullied or isolated.

So the next time you are furiously shaking a bottle of formula or pounding the mash, think about this:

1. What were your family's rules at the dinner table?
2. Were you made to clean your plate even if you weren't hungry?
3. How did your family or friends make you feel about your body?
4. How do you feel about your body now?

5. Was food used as a reward to make you do your homework or behave well in front of guests?
6. Was your family very 'food social'? Were there lots of guests, and activities which centered around the food cooked in your house?
7. How often did you celebrate with food?
8. Were you fed a lot? When were you allowed to feed yourself? At what age?

I'm not saying that any of the above is somehow wrong, but I am urging you to focus on what lessons you would like to take forward and which you would like to leave in the past. If you find yourself nodding at even one of these, I would encourage you to feed mindfully, nourish mindfully and be an active participant in the feeding process. These questions above should help you answer the biggest question of them all:

 What lessons do you want your child to learn about nutrition?

Take time to think about the nutritional lessons at the dinner table and not just nutrition itself. Because with lifestyle diseases linked to overeating or poor dietary patterns – like diabetes, obesity and heart disease (India is the diabetes capital of the world[1]) – you will realize that, with incorrect food habits, there is no happily ever after.

The End

Introduction to Solids
Age Six Months to Two Years

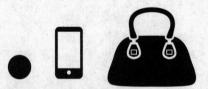

Comparative size of child's stomach between six months
and two years. Indicative.

The introduction of solids – from age six months to two years
– is a major milestone for you and for your baby. Her muscles

for chewing have been developed and her digestive system is now six months old, which is – believe it or not – how old the baby is as well. To celebrate this uncanny coincidence, people start the process of introducing solids to this hitherto purely liquid-ingesting baby. And they do this not only because the baby can now chew. 'Liquid' breakfasts, lunches and dinners – and all snacks in between – are no longer sufficient for your growing infant. Breast-milk nutrition needs to be supplemented and your skills at mashing food need to be complimented. But I digress.

How exactly would you know it is time to switch to solids? While no baby clock strikes at exactly six months to the hour – although wouldn't that have been nice? – there are some signs to look out for to see if your baby is giving you food for thought. But before introducing anything new at all, it is best to

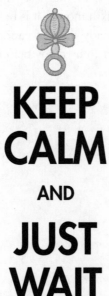

KEEP
CALM

AND

JUST
WAIT

Boldly going where your baby has not gone before is not an ideal strategy in these cases. Adding solids to a baby's diet before the six-month milestone has been linked to weight gain and adiposity (obesity) in both infancy and childhood. Early introduction of solids has also been associated with more incidences of colic, digestion problems and allergies.[1] Additionally, another reason for waiting is that the four to six-month period is a crucial one, where your little munchkin is developing her ability to chew as well as developing the enzymes that are needed for digestion; it pays to hold off the solids until these enzymes are completely formed. Before the age of four months babies have limited kidney function (or renal capacity), insufficient neuromuscular coordination and an underdeveloped gastrointestinal tract (GIT). Not the perfect recipe for solid foods, obviously.

Although waiting is the hardest when the clock in your head is striking the sixth month, it is best to see if your baby is developmentally ready to start eating solids, though it is extremely rare for her to be ready before time. You could do this by:

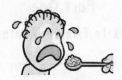

Looking out for her hand-eye coordination, so that she can look at the food, pick it up and put it in her mouth, all without assistance. You also need to check if the baby can open and close her mouth around a spoon.

Checking if she is able to move food to the back of her mouth using the up-and-down movements of the jaw. This can be done by using a small amount of mashed or pureed food. Babies who are not ready will show the 'tongue-thrust reflex', which will spit or reject foreign objects.

Placing her in a high chair and seeing if she can manage sitting up without your help. She needs to hold her head up unassisted and have good neck strength.

Don't mistake your baby's readiness to eat solids with other signs such as chewing her fists, waking up in the night when she otherwise sleeps through it or demanding extra milk feeds.[2] If you have identified the above, your baby is ready for solids and by that I mean pureed and mashed foods only. I have broken this chapter up into six to twelve months and twelve to twenty-four months because as communication skills evolve and your baby's likes become more pronounced, both the foods and the feeding techniques will change. As will the experience. For both you and your baby.

Part One

Six to Twelve Months

I. Eating or Learning to Eat?

Before I go into the difference
between eating and the more
active notion of learning to
eat, I just wanted to discuss
the concept of 'expectation'
because it is fundamental to the
business of feeding and child
nutrition in general, so bear
with me. I think the problem
with expectation, especially
those of the unrealistic kind,
is that it is entirely defined
by the one who is doing the
expecting. As the Expectors,
apart from expecting things
from themselves and pushing
from themselves and pushing

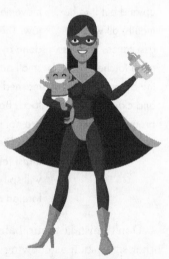

Expector, As Imagined
By Me

themselves to a relentless degree, parents also expect things
from the environment that would need to fall into place to
fulfil these expectations. But any parent who has been up
close and personal with breastfeeding would probably also be
up close and personal with the truth that parenting is pretty

much about expecting the unexpected. Unfortunately – or fortunately – please do remember, especially in this phase, that the only person you can control is you. Expect nothing from your baby.

Weaning off breast milk is also a bit misleading. My recommendation is that breastfeeding needs to continue as an adjunct to solids at this point, ideally till the baby is about ten to twelve months old. Even though the WHO recommends that breastfeeding continue for up to two years, as discussed earlier, this is best left to the discretion of the parent and is a conversation between mummy, baby and doctor. Do note that so long as you continue breastfeeding, your baby will still be protected from infections. So at the six to twelve-months mark, expect to continue breastfeeding, interspersed with feeding sessions of small solids, which will gradually increase in both quality and quantity.

Eating Versus Learning to Eat

There are two broad approaches to introducing solids and I thought it would be useful to outline the difference. The first approach is a common one. It includes spoon-feeding the baby with mashed and pureed foods after the age of six months when the parameters for solid feeding as mentioned earlier have been met. For a desperate want of a better phrase – and you'll know why the distinction is important soon enough – I have creatively called this approach 'Eating'.

However, in the second approach, 'Learning to Eat', you supervise the introduction of solid food to your baby. The operative word being 'introduction'. It is almost like a conversation that may go a bit like this:

> **'Hello food, meet baby.
> Baby, meet food.'**

As a parent, you don't want to dominate this conversation because both your baby and the solid food are strangers. Even though they don't know each other and don't even know what to do with each other, it is best to let them figure it out on their own. The conversation may as well be between two foreigners who don't speak the same language. When your baby reaches the age of six months, your job as a parent is to simply start that conversation. And leave them alone while you are at it. As a technique to get your baby used to solids, the second approach is something I think will work well.

This process of letting your baby discover solids on her own also has a name. It is called 'baby-led weaning' and is a technique developed by Gill Rapley. This approximately ten-year-old UK-born technique has proven to be immensely popular and has been adapted by different cultures all over the world. The key idea behind it is that instead of feeding the baby with a spoon, *you let the baby feed herself.* Even at the age of six months. This approach reminds me of a phrase I came across in a book I once read as a child, where the protagonist kept saying, 'What a capital idea!' as a way to express a good one. While this phrase doesn't seem to have too many takers, you seem to be a captive audience, so I thought I would reintroduce it: baby-led weaning is a capital idea.

The technique includes:

1. Creating an environment for the baby to feed herself by laying out the food in front of her.
2. Letting her touch, hold and discover the food on her own.
3. Not forcing her to eat or to play with the food.
4. Allowing her to give up when she wants to.
5. Supervising the process but not interfering unless there is an emergency.

The theory behind baby-led weaning is that if babies learn to crawl, walk and talk at their own pace, they can learn to eat at their own pace too. The operative word here is 'learn'. In baby-led weaning:

 Eating is not a physiological imperative for survival, but a skill that needs to be learnt.

With that crucial difference understood, parents can move from an active, on-the-frontline, in-the-thick-of-it role to a more passive, behind-the-scenes, I'll-catch-you-if-you-fall approach, which teaches a child much more than merely satiating her hunger. Baby-led weaning helps with motor development like hand-eye coordination, dexterity, chewing skills and the formation of good eating habits because, at this point, eating is not the main point, but the action of feeding is.

With spoon-feeding the child, a parent regulates just how much a child eats. While there are only good intentions behind this approach, it has to be acknowledged that not directly involving a child in monitoring her intake could lead her to lose her natural ability to self-regulate. Simply put:

 Spoon-fed children are more likely to become overweight than non-spoon-fed children, especially if satiety levels are not monitored.

It is simple human behaviour, no matter how little the human may be. If someone feeds us all the time, we won't put any thought into what and how we are eating. We would associate mealtimes with opening the mouth, closing it, chewing our food and opening it again.

 However, what I propose in the next section, 'How to Feed', is a combination of the two: spoon-feeding and baby-led weaning.

It is the take-the-middle-path, best-of-both-worlds approach which I find works best. It is a win-win situation. What the baby cannot manage by herself can be made up for by spoon-feeding.

And lastly, expect a mess during feeding time, especially with baby-led weaning. Your baby, floor, high chair and clothes could all be covered in the dish *du jour*, so do get used to picking out mashed apple from your hair or sofa. You can safeguard your interests by abandoning the idea of upholstery altogether. Or hair, if you like. But if you feel that you cannot imagine life bald and without cushion covers, don't forget to invest in a bib with long sleeves. And, if you are out shopping anyway, get one for your baby too.

II. How to Feed

From a lengthy distance.

I joke.

Since we are combining the baby-led weaning approach with spoon-feeding, I have devised a small mnemonic that I find is the quickest way to remember the 'How to Feed' part of this chapter. While as a parent, you will naturally evolve into your own feeding style and will probably develop a way of doing and remembering things, I thought I could start you off with the 5S approach, especially if this is your first experience with baby-led weaning.

1. **Sit.** Pull up a chair next to your baby's new and very important high chair (a high chair is in itself an exciting new milestone for both parent and baby, especially when the mother has been breastfeeding for so long). You can pick a time that works for you both. You can introduce new foods, for example, either in the morning or the afternoon. The reason for this is a practical one: if there is any allergic reaction to the food, it is easier to access your paediatrician during the day.

2. **Spread.** To teach your baby to feed herself, offer strips of boiled, soft food like the kind she can easily grasp but still eat. Don't introduce the option of spoon-feeding yet. Spread the food out and keep within easy reach. While I will get into what to eat (and what to avoid) in the six to twelve-months stage, for now, encourage her to touch the food by showing her, but resist the temptation to spoon-feed until you are sure she is done feeding herself.

3. **Supervise.** While you may think I am spelling out the obvious, I mean this in the context of hyper-supervision. Don't get too alarmed, panicky or stressed, although I know this can be hard for many – food is a foreign object in the child's mouth at this stage. Remember, the idea is to establish a fun and happy association with eating, not a stressed-out and unhappy one. If you choose to enjoy this, your baby will too.

4. **Sing.** Belt out a tune, dance or entertain; do whatever it takes to make mealtimes fun for the baby, especially at the introduction stage. This will help establish associations

of pleasure or entertainment with mealtimes and may have the added benefit of requiring less effort, in my belief, to bring her to the table later. And the definite upside of it is that you will almost always be rewarded with a heart-stopping smile or laugh for your effort.

5. **Spoon-feed.** Only spoon-feed when you are sure she is done with 'hand-feeding' herself and if you think she needs more. In other words, just because she has fed herself, it doesn't mean she has not done a good job. Try and gauge her fullness and then spoon-feed, if needed. I have elaborated further on quantities for this age group later in the book.

Needless to say, any solid food that will be spoon-fed to the baby, as mentioned before, needs to be mashed or pureed. The food must be soft enough to swallow and be accommodated in an infant's delicate digestive tract. It should be of the consistency that doesn't need chewing, so the baby can masticate with saliva and jaw movements and gulp down without a problem. Where the size of spoon-feeding helpings is concerned, start with teaspoons and then graduate to bigger helpings. Don't include small, hard bits of food like corn or peas, which can be a choking hazard.

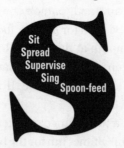

The 5S Approach

Whatever you do, don't give up even as you let your child take the lead. You may find that she is strongly against the concept of putting what she perceives to be foreign objects in her mouth. She may spit it out, cry and not want to try again. She has been used to breastfeeding so far, which needs comparatively less effort, so it may take her a little time to get used to this new sensation of solid food. As it is taking you. But to paraphrase celebrated author P.G. Wodehouse, you must plough 'doggedly on'.

The opposite of the 5S approach is, of course, what not to do when starting out in this crucial early phase. To that end, although it may be hard – and once again I speak from experience – think about:

1. **The Timing.** You know your baby best. There is a good time and a bad time for her to do new things. Your baby won't cooperate if she is tired or cranky.
2. **The Variety.** Try not to confuse her with too many options. It is best to introduce new foods once every four days, but sometimes foods can take as much as fifteen to twenty attempts to be accepted by your baby.
3. **The Gagging Reflex.** This is just her body's natural way of ensuring her safety. If she gags when she eats food which may be a bit tricky to swallow at this stage, don't worry too much about it.
4. **The Time.** Don't think about it too much. Give it ten to fifteen minutes at the very least, more if possible, to figure out if it was a successful feeding session. Else, try again at another time.
5. **The Safety.** Potential choking hazards include raisins, grapes (no matter how small), raw veggies and things which cannot be scarfed down by your baby at this stage.

I have given an indicative list (see the 'What Not to Feed' section) so that you are able to get the basic idea.

6. **The Signals.** Like I mentioned earlier, you know your baby best and you know her signs. If she reacts to your effort at introducing new foods by not eating or throwing it on the floor repeatedly, I think you can safely wrap up the proceedings and start the spoon-feeding section of the programme. If it looks like she has had enough, she probably has.

7. **The Emotion.** As a parent, it is very easy to get upset, frustrated or worried at these times. Don't make a big deal out of whether she is responding or not. If mealtimes are treated as a regular part of life, which they are, they will be seen like less of a mountain to climb.

Quantity at the Weaning Stage

How can you know that the child has had enough? You can begin with as little as one teaspoon. But this goes up slowly as the months go by. However, there is no hard and fast rule, per se. Quantities are a little subjective and depend on:[3]

1. **When the baby started on solids.** The earlier she starts, the more she eats at a later age. For example, a baby who started on solids at five months would eat more at six months than a baby who started solids at six months.

2. **What the food consistency is.** If the food is soft and diced, the baby will appear to eat less than one who is being spoon-fed.

3. **If the baby is unwell or teething.** If the poor little one is sickly, she may not want to eat as much. However, she will make up for this when she is feeling better

because that is when her appetite will come bouncing back.

4. **If your baby's growth spurt fluctuates.** Which it does. Babies will eat less post a growth spurt rather than during it.

III. What to Feed

For the more indecisive amongst you, breastfeeding may sometimes get you all nostalgic and teary-eyed for the good old times. One of the best things about that phase in your life was the limited amount of decisions you needed to make about what to feed your child. Planning her menu was literally restricted to your presence because *you* were the menu. So with solid food, when confronted with the conundrum about what to feed, how can this be simplified? Be made relatively stress-free? Keep in mind that at the introduction of the solids stage, you are not only required to start the baby on nutritionally rich, calorie-dense food, but you also have the responsibility of influencing her palate for life. So no pressure basically.

Here is a list of foods – specific to age – that you can gradually introduce her to as she discovers the world of solids:

Six to Seven Months (Both Months Inclusive)

Try and remember that even though I specified that you need to introduce a new food every four days, it can take your child up to ten to fifteen attempts to get used to a new kid on the block; so introduce a food every week, for example. Since it is the first introduction to solids, introduce calorie-dense foods, high in natural sugar, which are easier to digest than protein, carbs or fats. While you will be helping the child feed herself with the boiled, cut-in-strips version of the following, the below-mentioned foods are meant for spoon-feeding to give her what she doesn't feed herself. You could start off with the vitamins and minerals department:

Vitamins and Minerals

1. Stewed apple
2. Stewed pear
3. Stewed carrot
4. Mashed banana
5. Mashed chickoo
6. Mashed papaya
7. Mashed avocado
8. Mashed boiled sweet potato
9. Tomato and pumpkin soup
10. Stewed beetroot

Do I hear yummy in her tummy? Towards the end of the seventh month, you could also introduce the more-work-to-digest-but-nutritionally-necessary foods:

Protein, Carbs and Fats

1. Rice porridge
2. Ragi porridge
3. Lentil soup

Do note that nutritional gaps will have to be filled by breast milk. And as baby-led weaning will ensure that she eats something, stop spoon-feeding when she is full versus trying to see the bottom of an empty bowl.

Eight to Nine Months (Both Months Inclusive)

At the eight to nine-months stage, your baby would have had her first taste of chewing and swallowing solids, so this would be the right time to increase the lumpy texture in the purees. She will also start getting her first milk teeth. To celebrate this milestone, she can now sink her teeth into:

1. Ragi porridge with banana or chickoo
2. Sprouts and vegetable soup with mashed soft boiled rice
3. Oats porridge with stewed apples
4. Vegetable khichadi
5. Spinach moong dal with mashed soft boiled rice
6. Mixed vegetable rava upma
7. Idli with mixed vegetable soup

Ensure she tries to feed these herself first with the bits of food she can pick up, like idli or boiled vegetables, then spoon-feed. Or alternate spoon-feeding with self-feeding. Keep the baby-led weaning process going.

Ten to Twelve Months (Both Months Inclusive)

At the ten to twelve-months stage, when the child has more teeth, less mashed and chunkier food is what she needs to be seeing on the table. Now that she is older, you can further limit the spoon-feeding. See if she can feed herself:

1. Scrambled egg yolk with soft bread
   A note on eggs: only introduce egg yolks until the age of one. Egg whites have more allergens, so start her off on that only *after* her first birthday
2. Aloo paratha dipped in yogurt
3. Vegetable noodle soup
4. Paneer and vegetable paratha
5. Avocado mash with buttered bread
6. Soft dosa/uttappam or steamed idli with dal
7. Moong dal chillas with yogurt

8.   Oats and vegetable chilla
9.   Pasta with boiled vegetables
10.   Curd rice

Needless to say, the above are only indicative suggestions but if you find something more culturally relevant to you, by all means, go ahead. In the Appendix (page 207), the recipes for all of the above foods have been laid out in detail. But do note, however, that if your baby has any particularly unique health issues, your doctor would definitely be the best person to consult.

Introduction of Foods Versus Introduction of Flavours

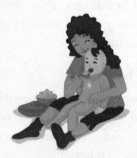

When I first started solids for my older daughter Ahaana, I followed the recipe to the T and after finishing, I took a bite. I emerged from this experience with profound respect. For her. For all babies. It was mashed khichadi lovingly prepared with my own two hands but up until that point, I had no idea what horror my two hands had the power of inflicting on a poor, defenceless nappy occupier. I mean, essentially, it was unsalted dal with unsalted rice and unsalted vegetables, mashed together to make unsalted khichadi, quite unpalatable to the adult palate. But it was eventually gulped down greedily – and may I add, appreciatively – by my baby. How was she eating it? If this meal was served at a restaurant, any self-respecting adult would be trolling their Facebook page by now. If you are not the best cook in the world, the beautiful thing about this six to twelve-months feeding phase is that your baby will never find out. Since you cannot, at this stage, add any seasoning like salt or sugar (you can add herbs and spices like turmeric and cinnamon), your job now is only to introduce foods and not flavours. Flavours – bitter, sweet, salty – are to be introduced later, after the age of one. Also, as an aside, *everything* cooked for the baby needs to be tasted by the caregiver or parent because you could have inadvertently added in a stale vegetable or salt, for example, without realizing it.

Staggered Breastfeeding and Solids Chart

Unless you have made the conscious decision of slowing down or stopping breastfeeding altogether, at the six-months stage you are essentially replacing one breast-milk (BM) feed at a time with solids. But if you are pondering over how to gently bring solids to the table, I thought it best to help you with, err, a table. I have mapped out a staggered feeding plan below, assuming your child feeds six times a day, sleeps about twelve hours a day and eats/drinks every two hours.

AGE	FEED 1	FEED 2	FEED 3	FEED 4	FEED 5	FEED 6
6-7 months (incl)	BM	Solids	BM	BM	BM	BM
8-9 months (incl)	BM	Solids	BM	Solids	BM/Solids	BM
10-12 months (incl)	BM	Solids	BM/Solids	Solids	BM	Solids

IV. What Not to Feed

Ah, the 'don'ts' list. The list of no-nos that parents should not say yes-yes to. Your paediatrician should give you a list along these lines but, as a nutritionist, I am just adding a few bits about other surprise hazards in case you don't have access to more information in this vein. This list doesn't just include what shouldn't be fed – keeping in mind your baby's delicate digestive plumbing – but also what could prove to cause allergic reactions.

Choking Hazards

While this is not an exhaustive list, you should get a general idea. Please avoid serving these foods to your infant ideally before she is at least *four* years or older, but do feel free to make your own interpretation:

1. **Chunky vegetables.** Raw vegetables and fruits (they should be ripe, soft or mashed), especially small cherry tomatoes.
2. **Seeds and nuts.** While seeds may not cause choking, they could get lodged in the airway, leading to an infection. So, if you are serving these to an older child, crush or finely chop them before serving.
3. **Dry fruits like raisins.** Small, but deadly.
4. **Popcorn.**
5. **Chunks of meat.**
6. **Sticky foods.** Peanut butter and caramel.
7. **Uncooked peas.**
8. **Corn.**
9. **Hard-boiled sweets and jellies.**
10. **Any chunk of food larger than a pea.**

Allergy Hazards

1. **Nuts.** Do wait even longer than one year of age if your family has a history of allergy to nuts.

2.   **Egg whites.**
3.   **Shellfish.** Prawn, crab, lobster and any other similar seafarers. As all good mammas tell their kids, don't be shellfish. Especially at this age.
4.   **Citrus fruits.** A surprising omission till the age of one. Citrus fruits are known to give babies a rash.
5.   **Strawberries.** Omitted till the age of one.
6.   **Chocolate.** The further you delay the introduction of chocolate, the better it is for your baby's teeth as well. Chocolate is also known to cause allergic reactions.

Other Hazards

1.   **Cow's milk.** While it seems innocuous, cow's milk contains more sodium and protein than a little body can digest, so it should be kept away from her before birthday number one. It also has the potential to cause allergies and reflux if introduced too early.
2.   **Unpasteurized milk.** Adults shouldn't be having this bacteria-filled food, so definitely not little babies with tiny tummies.
3.   **Honey.** It has been linked to botulism in babies.
4.   **Seafood.** Mercury levels can be dangerously high in fish like tuna, salmon and even sharks. Jaws will have to be closed for this one.
5.   **Tea and coffee.** Caffeine-rich beverages obstruct the absorption of calcium in your baby.
6.   **Carbonated drinks.** In a nutritionist's fantasy world, even adults should avoid drinks that contain such high levels of sugar, artificial flavour and sodium.
7.   **Salt.** There is enough sodium in the foods introduced to the baby and breast milk at this point. Added salt cannot be processed by them.

8. **Sugar.** There is a school of thought that believes introducing sugar too early could lead to toddlers growing into children with a marked preference for sugar. Why add it if you don't need to?

Part Two
Twelve to Twenty-Four Months

I. What to Expect

While I started this chapter urging you to expect nothing from your baby, I meant it pertained to that phase and that phase alone. The one where your bundle of joy was actually a bundle – all wrapped up in a cute little onesie, waiting for you to passively feed her when she couldn't herself. Now that her birth certificate celebrates its first birthday (people often forget that birth certificates have feelings too), I can tell you from first-hand experience (twice over) to expect the unexpected. As your bundle begins to unbundle, one of the biggest developments takes place during this phase for your child. I speak not, of course, of the slightly more intangible development of organs and digestive systems, but of the one big change that is a lot more fun for your baby: the development, or rather the discovery, of legs.

When your baby starts walking, no longer is she expected to be confined to or be in a place that bores her to tears. She is now free to vote with her feet. You can expect to be running after her as soon as you get her to sit down. Or just as your back is turned, you can expect to find her behind a refrigerator, dangerously close to the plug point or seeking the gentle charms of mud in a potted plant. You could also find her mulling over – and then acting upon – what would happen if she poked that porcelain elephant sitting peacefully for years in its habitat on the shelf. She is slowly discovering her world and there you are, right with her, slowly losing your mind.

Having said that, the twelve to twenty-four-months phase is incredibly exciting. It is truly wonderful to see your baby take her first steps. She is walking, she is talking, she is having 'conversations'. She is slowly stepping into this world: an exciting new milestone for both you and her. So when it comes to nutrition, like it was with baby-led weaning, continue to give her a little freedom at mealtimes because the one to two-year-old starts to assert her independence at the table. But when I say freedom I am mainly referring to you listening to her ability to understand her own feelings of fullness and satiety. So if she is feeling full or she is just not hungry, you may want to back off until she is ready to eat. There is also a developmental reason for this. Skipping meals is extremely common for toddlers as growth slows down during this phase. The galloping physical and mental development in the newborn and infant phase are now trotting along at a gentle canter. With growth settling down, appetites will also reduce.

Irrespective, nutrition should always be top priority. Expect kids to be too busy unloading the clean clothes from the washing machine and dragging them out to the living room than be concerned with mealtimes. It is also common for the one or two-year-old to not want to eat too much at one time. So, to circumvent this nutritional gap, you as an informed parent can fill it with the newest trick in your nutritional bag:

The Snack

The snack is the new addition to the diet and is that lovely between-meals solution which will help your child eat her way through this developmental phase. While I will get into exactly what to feed in the cleverly titled 'What to Feed' section, do remember that as a parent, continue to expose her to new foods and flavours.

II. What to Feed

At the age of twelve months and above, your child can start eating more 'normal' food and less baby food. At this stage, baby-led weaning still continues, breastfeeding stops and bottle-feeding – unless specified otherwise – is pretty much a thing of the past. Plates slowly begin to replace bottles. Your little baby is growing up.

After the age of one, your baby eats almost like the rest of the family and your role is to keep introducing more flavours, textures and, of course, quantity. You can also start adding more herbs, introduce salt, sugar (although I would try and delay sugar as much as possible) and other flavours. While sugar will never get fair representation in the court of any nutritionist worth her, err, salt, see the box 'Regulating Sweets for Your Sweet' (page 69) on how to introduce sugar in your baby's diet. I have also included some daily recommended allowances for salt later in this chapter.

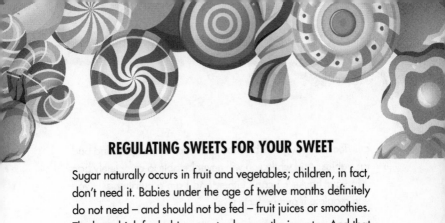

REGULATING SWEETS FOR YOUR SWEET

Sugar naturally occurs in fruit and vegetables; children, in fact, don't need it. Babies under the age of twelve months definitely do not need – and should not be fed – fruit juices or smoothies. The best drink for babies over twelve months is water. And that goes for all humans over twelve months too.

Avoid keeping your baby on pureed fruit for longer than indicated. Both fruit juices and purees strip the fruit of fibre, leaving primarily free sugar as the active ingredient. Free sugars can kick-start the process of tooth decay in delicate baby teeth. To further prevent decay, start your baby on a cup or beaker from the age of six months.

But it is the hidden sugars – lurking like big bad ogres in those bedtime stories – that you need to be truly careful about. Sugar sometimes masquerades as other ingredients on food labels like high fructose corn syrup, fructose, syrup, honey and cane sugar among more popular names, so keep a lookout for ingredients that you do not recognize. Other high-sugar items also include rusks, baby biscuits, candied fruit, and puddings. Purees and juices are even used to sweeten 'savoury' foods. The more sugar added to a baby's diet, the more she will develop a taste for it, the unhealthier it is and greater the chances of obesity. Sugar is bittersweet because the truth is so much darker than the soft and cuddly image it tries to send

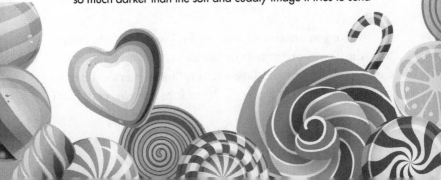

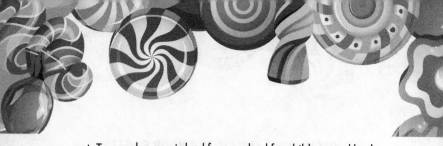

out. Too much sugar is bad for you, bad for children, and bad for babies. And while you will never be able to completely ban it in your house – I can't either, and I am a nutritionist – you can regulate it quite effectively.

The **maximum** recommended sugar allowances (you can serve less than this) for children and babies include:[4]

2 years = 3 tsp (13 grams a day)
3 years = 4 tsp (15 grams a day)
4-6 years = 5 tsp (19 grams a day)

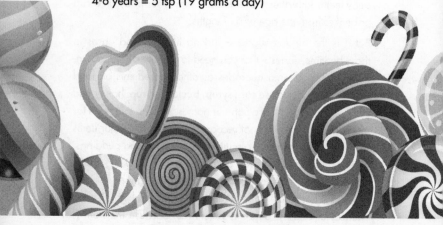

To give you an idea of what to feed your baby, do ensure that the five most important nutrients are accounted for: carbohydrates, protein, fats, vitamins and minerals. I like to call them the Five Fingers of Nutrition. Protein, carbs and fats are your *macro*nutrients and vitamins and minerals are your *micro*nutrients. Together, these five fingers of nutrition make a fist.

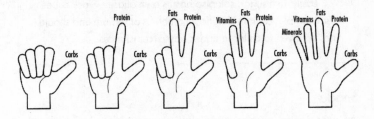

The Five Fingers of Nutrition, Dramatically Revealed

Your job is to make a nutritional fist and include all five in your child's daily diet. The following five fingers of nutrition have been designed for ages twelve to twenty-four months and include a few ideas on what they may like to eat. These are, of course, just broad guidelines and adaptation is very interpretive. Do note that fruits and vegetables belong to both the vitamins and minerals group, but I have assigned them to vitamins and minerals respectively for ease of reference.

NOT A PINCH OF SALT

Now that flavours are being introduced, it is best not to take salt with, err, a pinch of salt. Sodium, its active component, is hard for babies to absorb and their little systems can take only so much. The maximum daily salt allowance for children and babies is:

1-3 years = 2 grams (0.8 grams of sodium)

4-6 years = 3 grams (1.2 grams of sodium)

1 teaspoon = 5 grams[5]

Lastly, like sugar, salt also has its own aliases. Stock cubes, for example, contain significant amounts of sodium and should not be given to children under any circumstances.

Snacks

As mentioned earlier, toddlers have an uneven diet for the most part; healthy and timely snacks can fill up your little ball of energy and prevent her from getting so hungry that she becomes cranky. Snacks could also be a way to not only boost the intake of nutrients but also put your child in charge by using snack time as another opportunity to feed herself. When you are thinking 'snacks' for toddlers, think bite-sized finger foods like:

1. Wholegrain breakfast cereals like wheat or bajra puffs, quinoa puffs, makhanas and rice puffs
2. Khakras (do supervise the size of the piece they are eating)
3. Fresh fruit either cut into pieces or thinly sliced
4. Wholegrain crackers
5. Home-made breadsticks
6. Small cubes or slim sticks of cheese
7. Carrot sticks
8. Boiled eggs
9. Semi-crushed nuts to include almonds, cashews, walnuts or pistachios (but before that, see note on 'What Not to Feed')

VITAMINS

Fruits are an easy sell with toddlers and provide tons of important vitamins and minerals, along with fibre. You can never go wrong with seasonal fruits, and just about half a cup of cut fruit is enough to meet your baby's daily vitamin needs, even though you can give more. Provide citrus with Vitamin C-rich fruits like oranges, sweet lime and lime. Rich sources of Vitamin A include yellow fruits like mangoes and papayas.

MINERALS

Vegetables must be the main attraction in your baby's daily diet. They can be cooked or raw, depending on your baby's ability to ingest them. Vegetables are not only abundant in vitamins and minerals but also roughage, which keeps constipation at bay. To keep boredom at bay, however, serve fresh seasonal vegetables and get creative with the dishes.

FATS

Nuts like almonds, pistachios, cashews and walnuts are great sources of both protein and healthy fats, but do check the 'What Not to Feed' section for flagging off allergens. You can incorporate nuts, for example, by crushing them and adding to a dish. No whole nuts, please.

PROTEIN

A toddler's protein needs are met by drinking two glasses of milk (full-fat cow's milk) a day. Protein substitutes for milk include cheese, curd, paneer, chicken, eggs, fish, lentils. Experiment by giving well-cooked or semi-mashed chickpeas or kidney beans as finger food. This would also be a good time to introduce soyabean cutlets.

CARBS

Within carbs, grains are your best nutritional bet and every meal should have some kind of healthy grains. You can serve whole wheat, corn, rice, ragi, oats. Even bread, noodles or pasta, if your baby likes. Ragi can also be mixed with other foods.

FLUIDS

Your baby needs about a litre of fluids every day, but not necessarily from water alone. Milk is 90 per cent water and soups, juice and fruit all contain water too. But this would also be a good time to build the habit of drinking actual water. And while there is no need to track exactly how much is being consumed, do keep an eye on the number of times your baby urinates, fun though that job may be. Five to six times of clear urine means there is enough hydration but if the urine is darkish or not frequent enough, the fluid intake is low; something that needs to be watched out for.

Try to stick to a schedule even for snacks. As you probably already know, children are better with routine. This way, she will know what to expect from you.

And while you are acquainting your child with the idea of variety, learn from my story. When I first started weaning my older daughter, Ahaana, off breast milk, I was religious about ensuring she got her daily nutrition from khichadi, the dal-chawal-sabzi combo. It was the perfect food, I used to think to myself happily as I pounded the rice to feed her. What could go wrong? I mean, it was brimming with nutrients, including vitamins and minerals, and was a complete meal. Which sounded, well, sound except for one tiny detail.

I fed my poor daughter khichadi for one full year.
To this day, she hates it.
She is twelve now.

For me, my idea of variety was simply experimenting with the dal and the veggie for the day. In my mind, the variety box was ticked and she needed nothing else. Because I believed that baby food required little thought and creativity, I approached it as such. I would bump up the offering with a few spoons of dahi from time to time, but that was pretty much it. Till date, if I mix dal and rice, she won't eat it. She will eat the dal separately, the rice separately and the vegetables separately, but never all together. And while I am confident that she can make her mark in this world without being a khichadi lover, the important lesson that should be learnt from this is that just because your baby is a baby, it doesn't mean it is too early to introduce her to a smorgasbord of wonderful healthy things. You can serve the United Nations on your plate and that would be good for her. Let her eat India. Let her eat the world. Her journey to being a global citizen can start on her plate as early as possible.

Daily Dietary Requirements

As mentioned, nothing changes in the approach marked out for six to twelve-month-olds. But to make things more useful, I thought I would map out the total daily dietary requirements that your baby needs at this age. It is all very scientific and government-approved for Indian children, so 'it's all good', as my younger daughter says. This is for toddlers aged one to three years and it gradually increases to the higher end of the spectrum as your baby grows up.

Calories – 1000-1400 per day
Proteins – 16-20 grams
Calcium – 600 milligrams
Iron – 9 milligrams

Theoretically, you can go online and calculate how much protein one cup of dal has and so on, but I suggest you don't go overboard. Needless to say – but for some reason I still feel compelled to do so; must be a tic – your baby will get enough of the above with the right dietary choices you make for her, whether it is lean meats, veggies, fruits and milk. However, I have provided protein estimates in the mini chapter Rip Van Winkle (page 119), so do take a look if you like. Milk can be introduced after the age of one, as discussed earlier, but it must be pasteurized full-fat cow's milk. However, you do need to look out for one major possible dietary shortage that usually slips between the cracks: iron. The number of anaemic children – and adults – who come to my clinic are so many, it is scary. And as a nutritionist, I have seen it all.

BLOODY HELL

Anaemia occurs when the body does not have enough good, healthy red-blood cells. The role of these blood cells is an extremely important one: they transport oxygen to the tissues in the body. The role of iron, in turn, is to make red-blood cells. The deficiency of this very important mineral could lead to a condition called Iron Deficiency Anaemia. This condition commonly affects nine to twenty-four-month-olds and is a big health issue to flag off.

Babies are born with a store of iron but this gets depleted as they keep growing, since iron is needed for growth. Because of the baby's constant requirement for iron, parents need to watch out for iron deficiency in their infants as it can affect their physical, mental and behavioural development, and also lead to anaemia. As the iron levels keep going down, symptoms like irritability, breathlessness, craving strange foods (the condition is called pica), appetite reduction, weakness, tongue soreness, dizziness and headaches could start showing up.

Of course, iron levels can be restored to their optimum level through diet via iron-rich foods like apricots, lean white meats, eggs, dried beans, dals, soyabeans, spinach, kale, other green veggies, raisins, oatmeal and even prunes. Supplements can even be provided at the nod of your paediatrician, if your baby's test results don't look very encouraging.

Just a final note on cow's milk: babies who start drinking cow's milk too early (before the age of one) can also develop iron deficiency, as their bodies can't absorb it at that age. Which is why they should be started on full-fat cow's milk only after the age of one. The reason babies manage their iron levels while breastfeeding is because breast milk has just the right quantities of iron for your baby.[6]

Sample Schedule

As a lover of schedules and templates, I thought I would share the joy, so please do take a look at the table below. Three meals and three snacks a day is what I would nutritionally recommend for your toddler – assuming she sleeps twelve hours a day and goes to bed between 8 and 10 p.m. – with the snacks coming in mid-morning, mid-afternoon and post dinner, if needed. As mentioned earlier, it is important to maintain a schedule of both meals and snacks so that your baby will learn to expect food at certain times of the day.

Time	8 a.m.	10 a.m.	Noon	4 p.m.	6 p.m.	8 p.m.
Meal	Breakfast	Snack	Lunch	Snack	Dinner	Snack

Sample Menu

I also thought that I would map out a sample menu for a twelve to twenty-four-month-old baby to give you an idea of what her nutritional day should look like:

8 a.m. (Breakfast)	Ragi porridge or oats in milk (with crushed nuts and/or fruit)
10 a.m.	Two to four slices of apple or orange or banana or five to six cubes of watermelon or papaya
12 p.m. (Lunch)	Vegetable khichadi or sambhar rice or curd rice or dahi kadi and rice or soft cooked dosa/idli with sambhar
	Nap Time (assuming 2-4 p.m.)
4 p.m.	Milk with khakra/breakfast cereal or half a cheese/paneer sandwich

| 6 p.m. | Mixed vegetable soup or fruit |
| 8 p.m. (Dinner) | Soft cooked roti and vegetables and dal or vermicelli/rawa upma or dal paratha with curd or soft cooked dal chilla with grated carrots/spinach |

This is just indicative, of course, and menus will depend on cultural norms. We just need to ensure that nutrients – like various factions in any coalition government – are getting adequate representation. Also, do take your baby's nap time into consideration when you are planning her mealtimes. This is for your baby's comfort. And your mental safety.

III. What Not to Feed

At this point, the 'What Not to Feed' list should be short enough to be written in a paragraph because your baby would have been introduced to most foods by now. Having said that, there still lurk some common repeat offenders in the food environment, which should not be given to babies to eat. The choking hazards mentioned in the six to twelve-months section – like hard-boiled sweets, whole nuts, whole grapes and so on – still hold true for your baby, no matter what magic she wields with finger food in her high chair, so don't introduce these to twelve to twenty-four-month-olds either.

Also, do be on the lookout for allergic reactions when new foods are being introduced. The tendency of a child to develop allergies is higher if it runs in the family, so genes have an important role to play here. Even if allergic-type conditions like eczema or asthma exist among close family members, the tendency of the baby to develop an allergy will be higher. Sad, but true.

A Special Note on Nuts

In addition to some of your crazier extended family members or friends, nuts need to be introduced to your baby with extreme caution. Babies are classified into non-allergic and allergic, based not on their reactions to foods but their *families*. Non-allergic babies are defined as those who have no family history of food allergies or sensitivities while allergic babies, as you must have figured out by now, have somebody in the close family with an allergy. For non-allergic babies, some paediatricians sanction the inclusion of nuts into the diet before the age of twelve months, but that is usually rare. Most prescribe them after the age of one. For allergic babies, more caution is exercised. Paediatricians will recommend the introduction of nuts anywhere between twenty-four to thirty-six months, if not later. In these cases, waiting may also have the additional benefit of staving off the allergy entirely. Some doctors even go as far as waiting till after the age of seven, while some never recommend it at all. I would listen to your doctor with bated breath on this one, if I were you, because nut allergies can be debilitating at the very least. And fatal at the very worst.

I was in Dubai recently for an event and was catching up – and catching a ride – with a cousin and her little daughter, who was about one-and-a-half years old. My cousin, sitting in the front seat, told me to feed her child and I was happy to bond with her little girl. I opened her lunch box to find a few parathas. I was tearing them into small pieces for her to feed herself when suddenly our little interaction hit a bump. Frustrated by my feeding her pieces of paratha that she deemed too small for her, she proceeded to take the food from my hand and began eating big bites, furiously chomping

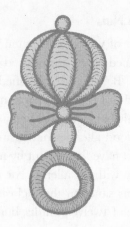

down and totally throwing my caution to the wind. When she was done, she put the corners of her paratha back in my hand and opened her palm to ask for the next one. She knew her level of hunger, made her own nutritional decisions and knew how to feed herself. Which is how it should be.

As a parent, there is something very special about watching your child graduate from breastfeeding to eating on her own. It is something that never gets old. By her second birthday, your baby can – and should – eat everything that the family does, controlling salt, spice, oil and sugar, of course. To that end, as she graduates to the 'big table', you are in a unique position of continuing to influence your baby's palate because only you or your spouse is in charge of making the decisions. The scenario that your one-year-old will call the *kirana* store and order chips, colas and chocolate to be home delivered is unlikely and, to that end, you become the gatekeeper of junk food; now it all comes down to what kind of gatekeeper you want to be. Your child will also not be exposed to too many food influences – like peers and the media – at such an age, so take advantage of this time to inculcate good eating habits which will set the stage for a healthy future.

THE ABCs OF INTRODUCTION TO SOLIDS

Chapter Summary

 When introducing solids to your infant, ensure that she is developmentally ready to do so. This would include seeing if she can sit up in a high chair without help, if she can use the up-and-down movements of her jaw and if she has hand-eye coordination, i.e., picking up the food and putting it in her mouth unassisted.

 There are two main techniques of feeding outlined in this book. The first is simply spoon-feeding the child. The second – called baby-led weaning – is teaching the child to wean off breast milk herself.

 In baby-led weaning, eating is not just done for survival. It is a skill that needs to be learnt.

 I believe a combination of baby-led weaning and spoon-feeding is the best approach to eating. Let the baby feed herself first. Spoon-feeding can help close any nutritional gaps.

 I have created the 5S approach for introducing solids, which includes sit, spread, supervise, sing, spoon-feed.

 When introducing solid foods, gradually increase the lumpiness of the purees and reduce the softening of foods as your baby develops her chewing skills over the course of a few months.

 Flavours – bitter, sweet, salty – are to be introduced post the age of one.

In the twelve to twenty-four-months age, your child is exploring her world as she has started to walk. Reciprocate her exploration by allowing her the ability to gauge her fullness.

 A one to two-year-old child may not finish her meals or may not always feel hungry at mealtimes. Supplement this nutritional gap by providing small snacks through the day: finger foods which she can 'feed' herself. Snacks should be scheduled so that your child knows to expect them.

 In food provided through the day, ensure that the five fingers of nutrition – protein, carbohydrates, fats, vitamins and minerals – are adequately represented.

 Babies aged nine to twenty-four months are particularly susceptible to low levels of iron. A deficiency of it could cause physical and developmental growth problems, and levels must therefore be monitored.

 Be very careful while introducing nuts to a baby's diet. They are highly allergenic. Babies whose parents or close family members are allergic have a higher chance of being allergic too.

Sleeping Beauty

Sleep and Child Nutrition

According to the story of *Sleeping Beauty*, a teenage princess had a curse put on her by a disgruntled witch who didn't make it to the guest list of the party for when the princess was born, and her birth in itself was a miracle that was granted by a frog, no less. It turns out that she was one heck of a powerful witch because this curse forced the princess and her family to sleep – now medically known as cryogenics – for about a hundred years at the age of fifteen. While she woke up later – kissed by a prince who seemed to be the only one equipped with GPS and a metaphorical chainsaw to cut through the dense vegetation that surrounded her pretty hard-to-locate castle, she emerged in history as the best-looking 115-year-old that ever lived. In the ultimate May-December wedding, she married this prince, younger than her by almost a century, with a face and body so amazingly intact that no anti-ageing brand of today could ever compete with the results, sponsored trial or no sponsored trial.

For the purposes of this book, the moral of Sleeping Beauty is that there is beauty in sleep. Even though one may not wake up a hundred years later looking like they are fifteen – indeed, one may not wake up at all – it cannot be denied that sleep is integral for health in adults. But in babies and children, it takes on a whole new dimension. Sleep is not just important, it is crucial for growth. This may not seem like it at first when your newborn is waking you up every few hours, but this will be more evident when she goes on to out-nap you on any sleep marathon that you may have ever participated in. A newborn needs anywhere between ten-and-a-half to eighteen hours of sleep every day in the first three months of her life, consistently crossing a double-digit sleep schedule all the way till the age of thirteen,[1] if not older. Here is what sleep looks like till your child is a teenager:

Age	Sleep Needed Per Day
Newborn-3 months	10.5-18 hours
4-11 months	9-12 hours
1-2 years	11-14 hours
3-5 years	11-13 hours
6-13 years	9-11 hours

That is a lot of zzzs, so why does it feel like neither parent nor baby is getting any sleep in the beginning? This is because the sleep-wake cycle – also called circadian rhythms – is regulated by light and dark. For the foetus, the windows were blacked out in her mother's womb, which is why the poor tiny newborn takes so much time to adjust when she is out the door. But what does this have to with nutrition, you ask? Well, growth is an intricate process, needing the help of hormones, which in turn will kick-start biological chain reactions in blood, muscles, bones and organs, regulated by light and dark. The human growth hormone is secreted by the pituitary gland and is a protein hormone. Many factors can tinker with its production like stress, exercise and nutrition. But in young children, what affects the production of the growth hormone most is sleep. Because while the growth hormone is discharged all through the day, the most intense burst of it is when your baby has just entered deep sleep.

But what has this got to with nutrition, you ask again? In addition to the growth hormone, there are other hormones that regulate appetite, satiety and metabolism and these include brothers-in-arms Leptin and Ghrelin (not to be confused with gremlin) as well as other hormones like Insulin and Cortisol. Sleep deprivation leads to dissention within the ranks of these hormones and their production is affected. Anything messing with these hormones leads to a tsunami of bad things that can happen and may lead to energy imbalances, obesity or weight gain. Simply put,

 Sleep deprivation can lead to obesity.

To corroborate the above, a mother-of-all-child-studies with a sample size of more than 9000 children was conducted, tracing their sleep journey from birth onwards. The results showed that those babies who were sleep-deprived at thirty months were more likely to be obese at the age of seven.[2] Sleeping babies are not just recharging their batteries and growing their bodies, they are staving off obesity.

Iron is another crucial nutrient needed for good sleep. If a child is struggling with insomnia, it could be a sign of iron deficiency. See box 'Bloody Hell' on page 75, for iron-boosting ideas. Also, if you notice your baby grinds her teeth while she sleeps, it could be a deficiency of zinc. This can be easily compensated via nuts and seeds, among other sources. You can supplement (or replace) these efforts with a supplement only on the recommendation of your paediatrician. Lastly, do note that with children:

 It is never about the quality of sleep. It is about the quantity, because quality of sleep is guaranteed.

When your child puts her head on the pillow, she will sleep well, so all you need to be concerned about is how many hours she is getting. And while there are many books on parenting which will give you more information on how to put a child to sleep – and sleep train if needed – this is best left to an expert in that domain. I just wanted to leave you with the thought that if you do see your child struggling with sleep, it is best not to sleep on it.

The End

Early Childhood Nutrition

Age Two to Five Years

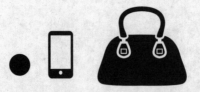

Comparative size of a baby's stomach between two and five years.
Indicative.

At the age of two to five years, the development of a child's palate, digestive system and taste buds also come head-to-head with the development of one more crucial element: an opinion. No longer can you unilaterally shove food in your child's mouth with minimal protest. He is now far more articulate in communicating his likes and dislikes with his own five-star rating system consisting of 'bleurghs', 'yucks' and 'ewws'. He has also begun the peaceful, lovely – and developmentally extremely important – journey of the terrible twos: where he tests both your boundaries and your patience. Having said that, at this age conversations with your baby are more complex, richer and deeper than they have been so far. He will ask you questions you probably can't answer only because you never thought to ask them yourself. Why *don't* cows wear shoes? *Do* rabbits get a haircut? Why *can't* you mix ketchup and milk? But God doesn't eat food either? All very good and valid points.

But this is when nutrition starts becoming truly participative for your child and not just you. At this age, you not only feed him whatever the family eats (making exceptions, of course, for too much spice, oil, salt and other contentious ingredients), you also ensure that nutrition is not just one-way: both you and your baby have nutritional 'jobs'[1] and the food department is no longer just yours. To that end, your, umm, KRAs include:

Job of the Child	Job of the Parent
To eat whatever is served	To choose and cook food under the most hygienic conditions

Job of the Child	Job of the Parent
To eat as much as he needs	To provide scheduled meals and snacks
To behave well during mealtimes	To teach mealtime behaviour and to abide by it themselves
To learn to eat foods the family eats	To make mealtimes pleasant and fun
To adhere to a routine	To train children not to eat other than when scheduled

If you looked carefully, you would have observed that the size of the 'briefcase' for both the baby and parent is the same. This is not because I am aesthetically obsessive – which I am and therefore not a fun person to be around when things, well, aren't – but it is to symbolize the fact that both baby and parent have a somewhat equal responsibility for nutrition; it must be shared between the two. This is the age where the child and the parent start to develop a nutritional partnership.

Yes, I am clinically sane. Today. I know that there is absolutely no chance in hell that you can take your adorable, waddling, spit-blowing cherub who may still have his bumsie in a onesie as a 'partner' in anything, but I guess the point of this exercise is to leave you with an idea. That:

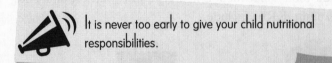

It is never too early to give your child nutritional responsibilities.

It is never too early to start teaching them mealtime etiquette. It is never too early to teach them to identify their own feelings of fullness. It is never too early to change our age-old attitudes of deriving satisfaction from a clean plate.

But like all things in life, you need to accept what you cannot change and have the wisdom to know the difference as you and your baby are both establishing your own boundaries. Learning to walk shouldn't mean walking all over you. Nutritional independence should not be confused with nutritional indiscipline. Let's megaphone this, shall we?

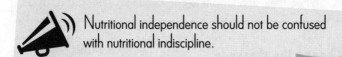

Nutritional independence should not be confused with nutritional indiscipline.

There is a very fine line between bolstering a child's independence (both nutritional and otherwise) and putting up with bad behaviour. And while saying no, throwing tantrums and refusing to follow instructions are all very normal – and vital – parts of human development at this age, it is best if you try to understand your child as quickly as possible. Find a strategy that works for both of you so you are able to help him benefit from the discipline of eating well. It will only be to his advantage in the end.

There is also a very fine line between a book on parenting and one on child nutrition. While I won't be expanding on table etiquette and behaviour unless it comes in the way of proper nutrition, the subsequent chapters in *Eat Delete Junior* will now be more concerned with the environment of eating and a child's responses to it. Using the techniques that have worked for me, I will elaborate on how to teach your child good nutrition.

Nutritional Guidelines
Two to Five Years

I. Change the Message

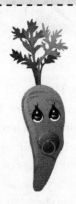

Once upon a time in a kingdom far, far away, a little prince or princess <insert correct gender here> was sitting at the table. His mummy prepared a yummy dinner for him and asked him to be a good boy. 'Finish all your food,' she lovingly told him as she patted his head. 'Don't leave the carrot <insert aspirational food here> alone. It gets lonely. You don't want anyone to be lonely, do you?' The good boy that he was, he listened to his mummy, finished the lonely carrot so quickly that his plate was shining like the moon. And because he listened to mummy, he never ever ignored the lonely vegetables again and lived a long healthy life <insert life aspiration here>. And he lived happily ever after. The End.

My Interpretation of a Sad, Lonely Carrot

One of the more effective ways to get through to toddlers and the odd adult, the story has been used by clever parents all over the world as a device to get their children to do what they want them to do: eat their veggies, clean their plates and do their little baby chores like picking up their toys. Invariably, the reward for doing so has some sort of existential benefit and marks the child's place in the world as one that has somehow become better because of said eating or cleaning. Dramatic though the above may be, I have often been even more dramatic in my quest to get my children to eat healthy food, but more on that later.

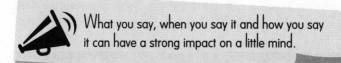

What you say, when you say it and how you say it can have a strong impact on a little mind.

As your children continue to flourish under your care, they take in everything they see. And whether you are aware of it or not, you are sending out signals about your relationship with food with every single utterance you make (see the mini-chapter 'Once Upon a Time' on page 43). You can lay the foundation for better nutritional habits by changing the conversation around food: the message, the tone and the intent. In 'The Lonely Carrot', the focus was to ensure that the child not only ate healthy but he also cleaned his plate, and *that* is the story which needs to change. Whatever your parenting style may be, whether it is indirectly weaving your message in a tale or barking direct orders like a benevolent military general:

You may need to focus on shifting the narrative around nutrition from unhealthy relationships to healthy relationships.

Something as innocuous as insisting that your child eat his veggies so he can go out and play immediately makes eating vegetables a form of punishment. Dessert then, by association, becomes a 'better food'. What are the other ways in which we unintentionally promote unhealthy nutritional relationships? Ooh, ooh! Pick me! Pick me! I can answer that. Thank you. For one, we do it through our daily instructions to our children. And here are a few ways we can change that:

UNHEALTHY INSTRUCTIONS	HEALTHY MESSAGES
'EAT THIS FOR MUMMA, PLEASE!' While innocent enough and very common, this message sends out that eating is a way to get approval and validation.	'THIS IS A MANGO. IT'S LIKE A STRAWBERRY, ONLY SWEETER.' This message points the child in the direction of appreciating the sensory qualities of food, thus making them more curious about the journey of eating itself. Eating then doesn't just focus on necessity, but discovery.
'WE MUST NEVER WASTE FOOD. ALWAYS FINISH WHAT IS ON YOUR PLATE.' Though it has its origins in the fact that there are many people around the world who don't get enough to eat, this message has been handed down to millions of children on this planet since the birth of the planet itself. What this conveys, of course, is that the feeling of fullness must be ignored. Wastage is of more importance than satiety.	'KNOCK, KNOCK, TUMMY. ARE YOU FULL?' As a lifelong fan of knock-knock jokes, I did feel the need to phrase it in the above way, but whatever you do, training a child to feel fullness is of paramount importance. Ask this question during or after every meal, and encourage him to come up with it first before you need to ask.

'YOU WON'T GET DESSERT TILL YOU FINISH YOUR VEGETABLES.' This inadvertently makes one particular food more aspirational than the rest.	'WHY DON'T WE TRY THESE VEGETABLES AGAIN? I'LL COOK THEM IN RICE AND MAKE YOU A YUMMY PULAO.' Instead of berating a child for not eating something, how about trying a more constructive approach? You will be sending out a message that food and mealtimes are not flashpoints of stress and unhappiness.
'IF YOU PICK UP YOUR TOYS, I'LL GIVE YOU CHOCOLATE.' This is classic reward-punishment behaviour and has been unconsciously used by many parents for decades as a way to teach their children to behave. Good child = 'good' food. Bad child = 'no' food. This will lead to a child rewarding themselves later in their lives with food for a job well done. Something we as adults occasionally also do.	"IF YOU PICK UP YOUR TOYS, YOU'RE A BIG BOY AND YOU'LL BE HELPING MUMMY.' Change the behaviour by changing the reward. What else is aspirational for your child? Being a 'grown-up'? Getting a gold star? Find something that motivates your child other than food alone.

Before you get all combative on me, I just wanted to point out that these examples are not a comment on your parenting, so try not to take it personally if you recognize yourself in them. If these seem to be ringing way too many bells, it probably just means that you have been raised to believe these things. And your parents before you. And their parents before them. Your own relationship with food is a complex and tricky one and can sometimes be tied to beliefs so old that it may seem intrinsically part of you. Don't worry about the ringing bells. Just stop the clanging and break the cycle.

And yes, it is easier said than done.

But change starts with you.

The dialogues are just examples of the signals you send out. Choose different vehicles such as stories, songs or the media – like cartoons or puppet shows – which support healthy nutritional choices and the message you want to send to your child. The moral of all these stories is that you have to:

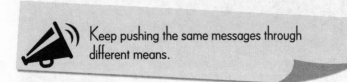

Keep pushing the same messages through different means.

II. Set an Example

The saddest part of being a parent is that it forces you to be a better person. Well, what if you don't want to be a better person? What if you like yourself just the way you are? A regular adult, with all flaws and bad habits, ungainly, with jagged edges. But alas, if we have children, bad habits like sitting all day in our pyjamas on Sunday is not to be. We have to get up and do something. We need to set an example because children at such tender ages pick up more than just colds. They are not only learning to talk but also need to learn to speak the language of nutrition. And you will have to talk the talk. Chat up a storm if you have to.

Eating with Your Child

At the age of two, your child has now probably graduated from a high chair to a booster seat. This would be a fantastic time to make him eat with the family at the big table. This will not only help him continue to develop his nutritional and social skills, but can also provide you with an excellent chance to set behaviours which your child can imitate. To that end, you can:

Focus. Turn off the TV, switch off the cell phone – pretend to, at least – and focus on the meal you are having with your family. Being distracted while eating not only leads to consuming more than you need, but it also means you are losing opportunities – no matter how small – to bond with your family and teaching your child to do the same. As your child grows older and gets wrapped up in his life, mealtimes will probably be one of the few focused opportunities in the day to communicate with him. If you treat mealtimes as sacred, he will learn to as well.

Experiment. Try new things and let your child watch you as you try exotic fruits and vegetables. Or even something non-exotic that you have been meaning to try, like eggs. Let him see you enjoy the nutritional wonders of kale, quinoa or spinach. Ideally, let him not see you spit it out if you don't.

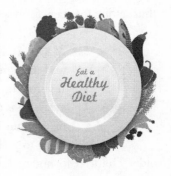

Share. Bring new foods to the table and share. Let your child eat what you are eating, barring, of course, any foods that children of that age are not allowed to eat. Break a piece of dim sum or tofu and give it to your child to taste. Pique his interest. Seeing you share will also encourage him to share his food with others.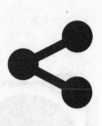

Engage. Engage your child in the cooking process. Making him mummy/daddy's little helper by enlisting his help in preparing small snacks and meals can really encourage him to get more excited about food and the process of preparing a meal, especially if he 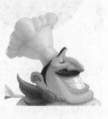 fusses while eating. He can, in this way, eat something he made with his own wittle hands. Also, ask your child to help with cleaning, wiping, setting the table and so on, thus setting the stage for responsibility and community eating.

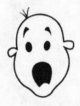 **Make it Happy.** As much as possible, try and make mealtimes positive and stress-free. Involve the little one in your conversations, even if it is to ask them what they really think of climate change; maybe they have got a bone to pick with the world too. Encourage older children to not make faces at the table if something they don't like is being served. Encourage the adults too, for that matter. Associating mealtimes with happiness and the relative absence of stress could really go a long way towards developing a positive association with mealtimes and, therefore, food.

Associating mealtimes with happiness and the relative absence of stress could go a long way towards developing a positive association with mealtimes and, therefore, food.

When my younger one, Amaira, started to eat at the big table, she began to notice that Mummy would eat a fresh salad with her dinner. Her eyes used to follow this plate from when it appeared to when it sat down on the table, a bit like at a tennis match. She didn't get a salad only because her meal was balanced, but she wanted one because her mother ate one. Before the next meal, she waddled all the way to the kitchen to ask for a salad of her own. Though my heart started doing cartwheels and a tear came to my eye, I realize that as a nutritionist, genuinely liking all the ghaas-phoos in the world can be a stretch for most parents, forget kids. Setting an example is, of course, not easy, especially when you are fussy yourself or notorious for refusing to share your food. But it all boils down to how committed you are to the process. And who knows, maybe – like so many parents – your child could teach you a thing or two? Or at least make you think a bit. I mean, why *can't* you mix ketchup and milk?

III. What to Feed

While this chapter, like the next few, will touch upon food ideas and portion sizes, the idea that you need the five fingers of nutrition to make a fist every day for the purpose of growth and development has now been established and is a

Working Things Out

Exercises for kids

Children need to exercise. An hour at least every day. In fact, they should not be sitting still for more than one hour at any time of the day with the exception of naptime or when they sleep at night. Exercise – while sounding too officious for your toddler – could mean simple, fun things like riding a tricycle, swimming, going to playgrounds and parks, dancing up a storm, jumping, hopping or simply walking; anything that gets them moving. Any good, consistent activity goes a long way in helping your child expend excess energy, leaving him with the ability to be more focused on learning activities, resulting in sounder, better sleep at night. See what you can do about limiting or completely avoiding time in front of the TV and iPads.

principle that is vitally and incredibly relevant all the way up to adulthood. You should make a five-finger nutrition fist, no matter how old you are. However, where portion sizes are concerned, you should feed your child approximately half of what an adult would eat. I have outlined the servings sizes needed per day for children in the two to five age group, but these are only indicative. As I still like to do nothing better than curl up with a glass of water and cozy up to a table, here you go, for your viewing pleasure, another table:

FOOD	TWO-YEAR-OLDS	THREE-YEAR-OLDS	FOUR TO FIVE-YEAR-OLDS	SERVING SIZE
Fruits	1 serving	1-1.5 servings	1-1.5 servings	1 serving of fruit = 1 medium apple: slices or cubes or 1 medium banana: slices or mashed or 7 large strawberries or 1 bowl of watermelon: cubes or balls or 1 medium orange: slices
Vegetables	1 serving	1-1.5 servings	1.5-2 servings	1 serving of vegetables = 1 bowl raw leafy greens or 1/2 bowl of carrots/bottle gourd/potatoes: mashed, sliced or chopped or 1 bowl vegetable soup or 2 tablespoons of avocado 1 bowl = 150gms

FOOD	TWO-YEAR-OLDS	THREE-YEAR-OLDS	FOUR TO FIVE-YEAR-OLDS	SERVING SIZE
Cereal	3 servings	4-5 servings	4-5 servings	1 serving of cereal = 1 slice of bread or 1 roti (6" diameter) or 1/2 bowl of cooked rice/poha/upma or pasta/noodles
Protein	2 servings	2.5 servings	3 servings	1 serving of protein = 1 egg or 1/2 bowl of cooked dals/pulses/sprouts or 30 grams of raw chicken/fish or chicken nuggets – 3
Dairy Low Fat or Fat Free	2 cups (1 cup = 240 ml)	2.5 cups	2.5 cups	1 serving of dairy = 1 cup milk or 3-4 cubes of cottage cheese/paneer or 1 bowl of yogurt or processed cheese – 1 slice/1 triangle or string

Do note, as mentioned earlier, that since children at this age need about eleven to fourteen hours of sleep, including naps, it is best to plan mealtimes around sleep schedules if you want your meals to go down well. Offer only water to drink with food, keeping in mind that your child is watching what you drink. So if you want your child's teeth to be cola-free, keep your table cola-free. Also, the other non-meal drink options are non-fat or low-fat milk because there is a general consensus that after the age of two years, such kind of milk is nutritionally apt for them. Please avoid giving fruit juices, fruit drinks or sports drinks. They are *loaded* with sugar and have no – or very scant – nutritional value to speak of. Also, don't be alarmed if your child doesn't eat the amount of food prescribed for his age. He could eat more or less, depending extensively on his growth spurts. Appetites can also vary from day to day, so take a deep breath and do some pranayama if this is stressing you out. In general, taller and more active children will eat larger portions of some foods than smaller and less active children. But if you feel your child is being unusually fussy and you seem to be walking on eggshells more than peeling them, you may have on your hands a picky eater.

IV. When They Don't Want to Eat

You put a plate down on the table. You just lost about thirty minutes of your life cutting hearts out of apples for the first time with fingers you never thought were nimble. Satisfied that you have indeed learnt something new and there is a crown in your future with the words 'Parent of the Year', you excitedly put the plate down in front of the apple of your eye, expecting him to start chomping it down. The apple that is, of course, not your eye. But instead of seeing him look up at you with stars in his eyes, he winds up looking a bit like a grouchy food critic about to strip your Michelin-starred restaurant of its only star because the entrée was a piece of resistance.

Nope. No stars. Not one.

Subsequent attempts of placing hearts, stars, moons and indeed the entire cast of *Peppa Pig* in front of him seem to fail. All you seem to get in return is a child disinterested in either eating the entire meal or parts of it. Maybe the pasta is too sludgy or the bread is too 'bready'. Sometimes it is even textures and not just flavours which can genuinely put your child off. He is not doing it to get back at you. He has just entered a brand new phase. Because, you know, development.

The two to five age group is when picky eating starts to rear its picky head. My advice would be to choose the option where you can hold on to your sanity because you will probably lose it anyway when your kids hit puberty. As a way to help you deal with this phase, let's remember to:

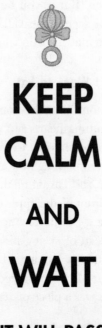

KEEP

CALM

AND

WAIT

IT WILL PASS

Picky eating is a phase – only in rare cases is it not and could be symptomatic of something deeper; see The Princess and the Pea: The Pathology of Fuss (page 116) – and, like all phases, it will pass. You just need to do the best you can. Luckily, your fairy godmother – me – is here to provide you with tricks on how to handle the trickier parts of this phase. If your child is essentially driving you crazy and is a bundle of energy bouncing off the walls, it means all is well. So long as your child is energetic, bright, engaged, alert, is at a healthy weight and seems to be growing in line with his age, it means he is feeding himself properly and is getting what he needs even if he leaves his plate half-empty sometimes (or half-full, if you are an optimist).

But **nutrition is nutrition** and, as a nutritionist, I have embroidered this phrase on my pillows and guest towels. Okay, I haven't, but I would be aghast at letting any child roam about entirely free without trying to plug nutritional gaps, especially if your child is not energetic, bright or engaged and picky eating is affecting him. So here is what you can do to deal with picky eaters:

The Gritted Teeth   The I-Don't-Wanna   The Why-are-You-Doing-This-to-Me   The Shock-and-Awe   The Whatevs   The Meltdown

A Mini Spectrum of Picky-Eater Expressions

You can start by taking your picky eater grocery shopping with you. One, let them <u>help you select healthy foods</u>, thereby increasing their ownership of what they eat. If they picked it out, they must eat it, right? Two, you could also ask for their <u>help in meal preparation</u>, which will bring them closer to what they are eating, making them far more involved in the process. Children are more likely to look forward to eating something they made. Three, <u>introduce all new foods at the start of the meal</u>. This is when your child is at his hungriest and will be more willing to sample them. Four, see <u>if your child likes his food mixed or separated</u>. There are two kinds of people in this world, according to me: those who like their food all mixed up into one nebulous dish, and those who like to keep all the components of their meal separate. Dal is in the 'dal area', rice is in the 'rice area' and so on. These kinds of eaters ensure, to quote Rudyard Kipling, that 'never the twain shall meet'. My eldest is the non-mixing kind of person and will gingerly eat everything separately, so the only time the twain will ever deign to meet will be when she chews it. My younger one is not so twain-ey, preferring a more abstract-art approach to nutrition. For children who want things separate, it can be a character trait, so do select plates which have sections for them to pick and choose. Five, <u>offer your child some choices</u> in what he is about to eat. It could be a choice presented between two vegetables or protein, more to give your child a greater feeling of control over the process. Six, <u>wait</u>. Sometimes he just may not be hungry or want something else (read: sweet) instead. Put it away and bring it back when he asks for food, presenting him with the options he passed up on earlier. Seven, name a food. Needless to say, name it after your child. A fruit dish could simply be called Arjun's Apple. Cut it in the way Arjun likes it, getting him more excited about the process. Eight, get them to expend their energy. Encourage them to play before mealtimes. It will take care of some of the restlessness that may interfere with their ability to eat well. Nine, set an example. As discussed earlier, expect them to try new foods only if you do. Make a habit of introducing and sharing new foods at the table. If he sees you eating – and liking – healthy new foods, chances are that he will follow in your footsteps. Ten, never let your mother or mother-in-law whip up his favourite meal as a substitute for not eating what is served. Otherwise known as let-my-poor-grandchild-eat-his-favourite-aloo-paratha or the something-is-better-than-nothing approach.

The Fun Healthy Food Handbook

The Fun Healthy Food Handbook has a few shortcuts to making healthy food more attractive to your two to five-year old. Visual references have also been provided in colour in the Appendix. Also, don't forget to adjust portions as per your child's recommended serving. The vegetables should be soft and cut into small pieces so as to not become a choking hazard.

Mickey-Mouse-Shaped Rotis

Experiment with rotis that are made in different shapes, like Mickey Mouse. I say Mickey Mouse because that is the shape

I get with rotis after I originally aim to get a perfect circle. But you get the idea. On this Mouse, you can spread a layer of thick dal as the base and place dry-cooked, or even slightly mashed veggies which are the eyes, nose and mouth.

Butterfly Sandwich

Use circular cookie cutters in two different sizes to make butterfly sandwiches (with desired filling), adding appropriately sliced carrots and cucumbers to bring the butterfly to life. Small flower-shaped cookie cutters can be used to make flowers out of thinly sliced vegetables. Make coriander 'stems' and a grape 'caterpillar' to finish.

Rice Star

To make this celestial dish, first spread some rice out on a plate. Using a star-shaped cookie cutter, cut out a star shape and discard the rest. Put a blob of yellow dal which can be the sun and sprinkle some veggies to make smaller 'stars'.

Melon Magic

As you may have guessed by now, scoopers or cookie cutters in exciting shapes will be part of your arsenal to combat disinterest in what is being served. You can use them to cut watermelon or musk melon in child-friendly shapes like hearts and stars. Or even a sun.

Bunny Cutlets

While it sounds a little suspicious, this is actually nothing but a mixed vegetable cutlet decorated like a bunny with pieces of vegetables to make the eyes and the nose. To this, add carrot sticks as ears and a little bit of cheese as the bunny's teeth.

The Kid Pizza

Involve your child in the cooking process by asking him to create his own pizza. Let him exercise his creativity by 'decorating' his pizza with vegetables, chicken cubes, paneer or cheese. Or all of the above, if he likes it.

To Further Increase Consumption of Healthy Foods, Try:

1. Adding egg white to the atta dough
2. Diluting dosa batter with egg whites for thicker dosas
3. Adding cheese in the dosa to enhance flavour
4. Kneading atta with cooked dal or bhaji, giving them different names like rainbow rotis.
5. Serving no-sugar-added fruit custard

Vegetables are extremely important for the growth and development of your two to five-year-old and have tonnes of nutrients which are critical to get your child to the next level. It is important that you try to bung them in (see The Fun Healthy Food Handbook on page 107) more creative ways if the path most trodden is finding few takers. Of course, if your child isn't getting enough, your paediatrician will suggest a course that derives these nutrients from other sources. But as I mentioned earlier:

If your kid is a picky eater but is growing — according to your paediatrician — and is active, you have nothing to worry about from the nutritional standpoint.

New foods can take time to become a part of your child's diet and it is best not to give up administering them. At first, if you don't succeed, ~~cry~~ try again. I mean, think about it: this is their first introduction to so many foods with varying textures and tastes. It may even be their first introduction to a flavour like bitter, for example. Have empathy for their palate and don't nip your attempts in the (taste) bud. It is an established fact that the average human being establishes his eating habits at the tender ages of two or three. So a vegetable-eating child will have a far higher probability of growing into a vegetable-eating adult. But so will a cola, fries, chips, junk-food-loving child grow into a junk-loving adult. But keep it going. You need to trust your child and believe with all your heart that it will be all right in the end.

THE ABCs OF EARLY CHILDHOOD NUTRITION: TWO TO FIVE YEARS

Chapter Summary

In the two to five age group, both the parent and the child have nutritional responsibilities and it is never too early to teach that to your child. Treat them like a nutritional 'partner'.

However, since this is the age where children enter the phase of the terrible twos, it is important to understand the difference between nutritional independence and nutritional indiscipline. Discipline is sure to benefit your child in the end.

Change the behaviour by changing the message. What you say, when you say it and how you say it can all deeply affect your child. But first, don't forget to consciously examine your own relationship with food. You will be surprised by what lessons you may be inadvertently passing on.

Sometimes attitudes towards food can be deep-rooted and generational, so don't expect a quick fix.

This is the age when a child begins to eat with the family. The best way to teach him good nutritional examples is by setting good ones yourself. Make mealtimes sacred and encourage experimentation. Other ways to set an example is to engage him in both conversation and meal preparation, share new foods and keep the environment happy and positive.

Children of this age need to sleep for about eleven to fourteen hours, which includes naps. The best way to get the most out of mealtimes is to schedule them around sleep times. Feed them about half the size of an adult portion. Don't forget to account for all the five nutrients, i.e., the five fingers of nutrition.

Only water should be provided at mealtimes for children to drink. Other options include low-fat or non-fat milk. Do not give them fruit juices, fruit drinks or sports drinks. These are loaded with sugar and have little – or no – nutritional value.

The age group of two to five is also one where picky eating rears its head. It is a phase and – unless there is an underlying condition – it will pass. However, you can combat this phase using the techniques outlined in this chapter. These include taking your child grocery shopping, asking for his help in meal preparation, introducing new foods at the start of the meal, keeping foods on the plate separate if he doesn't like it, serving the same food at another time if he is being fussy, naming a dish after him, setting an example for him, getting him to expend his energy and offering a few meal choices, but between healthy foods.

Children at this age must exercise for at least sixty minutes a day.

The Little Mermaid

A Special Note on Water

When solids start to make their entrance into your child's diet, water needs to start paying regular visits too. Even mild dehydration – as little as weight loss of 1 per cent of body weight – could temporarily impair concentration and mental performance.[1] Other studies[2] draw links *between* adequate hydration and visual attention, short-term memory and fine motor skills (for example, handwriting). Water also brilliantly helps with the transportation of nutrients to cells, the lubrication of muscles and joints, the regulation of body temperature as well as blood circulation and digestion.

This may come as a bit of a surprise but children need more water *in proportion to their body size* than adults do. This is because the need for water depends on metabolism and the quicker the metabolism, greater the requirement for water. So how much water do children need? Well, the prescribed age and gender adequate intake (AI) for water is as follows:

Age[3]	Prescribed AI
0–6 months	0.7 litres/day, assumed to be from breast milk
7–12 months	0.8 litres/day, assumed to be from breast milk, as well as solids and other beverages
1–3 years	1.3 litres/day

Age	Prescribed AI
3–8 years	1.7 litres/day
9–13 years (boys)	2.4 litres/day
9–13 years (girls)	2.1 litres/day
14–18 years (boys)	3.3 litres/day
14–18 years (girls)	2.3 litres/day

Even though it is an essential propellant of child development, most children don't drink as much water as they need. There could be a few reasons for this. For starters, children have to depend on their parents or caretakers for water; they cannot reach out for it on their own. Second, they are still too little to identify feelings of thirst, which makes them especially vulnerable to dehydration. A possible third reason could be the wonderfully vague they-simply-don't-like-it.

Either way, like it or not, they have to. So how can you ensure that they do? If your child doesn't take to hydrating as a fish takes to, well, water, you can:

1. Make it exciting for them using fun bottles and silly straws.
2. Use reverse psychology: don't finish it — just take one sip, you warn. Then watch them drain the cup.
3. Make a game out of it while teaching them the 'pee test'. Clear urine means that they are 'winning'. Though try to make sure they don't announce the results in front of guests.

4. After the silliness of the bottles and straws wears off, which it inevitably will, you may want to entice them with a beaker or a decanter that has a small tap. Ask them to serve themselves when they need it. This teaches them responsibility and independence. And just to show that independence, they drink and then drink some more.

5. Weather permitting and if your child is not unwell, freeze some berries or add frozen fruit cubes to the water. This makes it so much more exciting to drink now.

6. For older, school-going children, mark the bottle with the time – 10 a.m., 2 p.m. etc. – so they know how much water to finish and by when. Since there is a link between water and class performance, this could actually be a very important trick.

7. Be a water baby yourself. Set an example by drinking lots of water and make references to feeling better or worse without it.

8. Hydrate with food. This is a smart, ingenious way to include more water in your child's diet, which involves feeding them fruits and veggies which are high in water. These include strawberries (after the appropriate age), blueberries, celery, cucumber, tomatoes and watermelon, to name a few.

The End

The Princess and the Pea

The Pathology of Fuss

In *The Princess and the Pea*, the protagonist was – unbeknownst to her – put through a test that would determine whether she was royal or not, orchestrated by the placement of a pea under about twenty mattresses. If she 'felt' the pea while sleeping, she was a princess. While she passed the test and will probably go on to be blacklisted by most hotels on account of her inability to find a room that makes her happy, the larger point is that extreme sensitivity could be a sign of something bigger. And even if you have already ascertained your child is a royal, what I am trying to say is if your offspring is pushing away most of his food during mealtimes, you may want to consider it to be a symptom of an underlying condition. Not all pickiness is created equal.

Nutritional problems are of two kinds – sometimes called the binary law of nutrition[1] – and the law goes a bit like this: either something is irritating your child or something is missing from his diet. In other words, there is either something there that shouldn't be, or something that should be there and isn't. While you are re-reading that last sentence, let me take on some common situations which could mean that your child could need a doctor and is not just being fussy. Colon impaction, acid reflux, gluten intolerance and lactose intolerance are all conditions which have nothing to do with pickiness but more to do with genuine, tangible, negative reactions to food. In other words, maybe your child is pushing

116

away the roti not because he is being picky but because his system cannot handle it. Eating wheat makes him feel bad and he doesn't know why.

Usually, if it is a condition – although you may have to check with your paediatrician – other symptoms may coexist with the symptom of pickiness. Symptoms of gluten intolerance, for example, include vomiting, diarrhoea, constipation, stomach ache, weight loss, mood swings and irritability.[2] So a picky eater who seems to be an angel one moment and Satan another could warrant a closer look at his diet. Similarly, lactose intolerance could translate into stomach cramps, diarrhoea and gas[3] for a hitherto healthy child who just seemed to be enjoying ice cream earlier that day.

And it is not only restricted to food irritants. A deceptively innocuous deficiency of zinc could alter a child's reception and experience of food. Low levels of zinc have been associated with either a complete loss or a sense of alteration of smell and taste to the point that even normal, regular foods could be unpleasant or strange to taste. Maybe he is pushing his plate away because his sense of taste has been altered.

Sometimes the ability of a child to eat could also be impaired. Symptoms include too much drooling, not graduating beyond mushy food, bad breath, too much time taken to eat, frequent gagging or vomiting, continuous complaints of stomach pain, or the absolute refusal to touch or sit near new foods.[4] While this would be a more advanced medical condition, I wanted to establish the notion that sometimes, there can be much more than what meets the eye.

Kelly Dorfman has come up with a wonderful way to help picky eaters include more variety in their diet. Called the E.A.T method, this technique helps expand a child's diet. You could start by:

E: Eliminating irritants. Whether it is gluten or dairy or anything else, first find out – with the help of a doctor or nutritionist – if something is indeed bothering your child nutritionally. Then remove it entirely from their diet.

A: Add one new food at a time. If you would like to expand your child's palate, one new food can be introduced every day like carrot or bottle gourd, if your child is eating too few vegetables. Add only one item each time though.

T: Try a bite of the food every night for two weeks. Encourage your offspring to be a sport and just try one bite. Over time, it will not be so hard for him to start tolerating – if not loving – the new food.

Children can be trained to expand their diets. Even if the apple of your eye isn't a picky eater, you can always try new ways to get him to eat better food and with it, get better nourishment.

The End

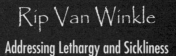

Rip Van Winkle

Addressing Lethargy and Sickliness

It is somewhat of an exaggeration to compare lethargic or sickly children with someone who napped for twenty years like Rip Van Winkle, but the point here is simply to shine a little light on why some children are more energetic than others. Of course, while your paediatrician should be your first port of call to ascertain if your child is suffering from a particular affliction – lethargy or sickliness could be a symptom of any number of conditions – I thought I could outline some nutritional reasons that may be responsible for slowing your child down physically.

Lack of Protein

Proteins are the ultimate building blocks which contain amino acids that help fight diseases, produce hormones and enzymes, repair a tissue here, build a bone there, transport nutrients, and are essential growth propellers that boost your little one to not-so-little-anymore. Quality, of course, is as important as quantity so lean protein like eggs, fish and white meats like chicken and turkey, dals, soyabean and quinoa would be the best weapons of protein dissemination as opposed to red meat or other high-fat sources. But if protein brings so much to the table, a shortage or absence of it may mean that muscles are not being repaired as quickly or other functions that need this macronutrient are being compromised, which could lead to your child not feeling as energetic or as good. Take a look and see if your child is getting enough:[1]

Age	Grams of Protein Per Day
1-3 years	16.7
4-6 years	20.1
7-9 years	29.5
10-12 years (boys)	39.9
10-12 years (girls)	40.4
13-15 years (boys)	54.3
13-15 years (girls)	51.9

Well, the above is all well and good, you say, but how does this information help you? To that end, I thought I could give you a clearer idea by indicating the protein content of a few common foods:

1. One egg = 6 grams of protein

2. Fish (100 grams) = 22-25 grams of protein

3. Soyabean (100 grams) = 43 grams of protein

4. Dal (100 grams) = 20-24 grams of protein

Lack of Vitamin C

A fantastic immunity booster, Vitamin C, is a vital part of making sure your child doesn't need too many sick days. While the amount of Vitamin C in the mother's milk is enough for a child who is still being breastfed (till the age of one), the following are the Vitamin C requirements for children aged one and over:[2]

Age	Mg of Vitamin C/Day
1-3 years	40
4-6 years	40
7-9 years	40
10-12 years (boys)	40
10-12 years (girls)	40
13-15 years (boys)	40
13-15 years (girls)	40

Food sources of Vitamin C include citrus fruits like oranges, red peppers, kale, broccoli, strawberries, amla, kiwi and grapefruit. To help you estimate quantities, one medium orange has about 70 mg of Vitamin C, one medium guava has about 206 mg and one medium mango has about 76 mg. Also don't forget to check in with your paediatrician from time to time, who may just recommend supplements.

Lack of Vitamin B12

Vitamin B12 not only affects immunity but also greatly impacts speed of recovery. Nutritionally however, B12 is a little tricky to find in a vegetarian diet because it is usually found primarily in animal foods – including dairy and eggs. Prescribing B12 supplements is medical territory so it is better to give your child a doctor-approved B12 supplement to ensure that proper levels of this vital vitamin are being

Lack of Zinc

Children are particularly susceptible to a deficiency of zinc, so take that into consideration when cooking for them. Zinc impacts the production of white-blood cells and with it, immunity. You can find zinc in certain nuts, poultry, beans, whole grains and dairy products. Certain breakfast cereals and foods are also fortified with this mineral.

If the problem isn't nutritional, your paediatrician will be the one to confirm that it isn't. Either way, it never hurts to eat healthy and work towards boosting immunity, no matter how your child feels.

The End

Older Child Nutrition
Age Six to Nine Years

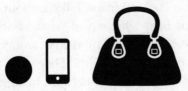

Comparative size of a child's stomach between six and
nine years. Indicative.

The best way I can explain nutrition at this age is by using the
metaphor I used at the very start of this book, the one where

you dress up all nicely and step out only to have a passing vehicle splash dirty ditchwater all over you. Up until this point, you have done your job. You've set a saintly example of healthy eating, kept the family environment positive at the dining table – even if you want to bash one over your spouse's head – and have gently coaxed, cajoled and, sometimes, sneakily included more vegetables in your little one's diet. So far it is all working brilliantly according to plan, Sherlock, but suddenly, it is no longer elementary. Like the mother of all ditchwater-splashes, some of your hard work may soon be undone. There is a new fix in the mix now: peers.

 The six to nine age group is a new phase of independence for your child.

Friendships become deeper, and your child's social circle rivals yours. Social skills are a must alongside other subjects and many opportunities to interact – and eat – arise like class picnics, play dates and group activities. Peer influence now kicks in full throttle. Children come home, dragging their schoolbags behind them, talking about who got what in their lunch box, who served what at which birthday, whose cake was better than theirs, among many other similar socio-political minefields. They want to be the best, even when it comes to food, because being the best is the discourse they are often exposed to (my feelings about this discourse notwithstanding).

By six to nine years of age, eating habits have been more

Because of peer influence, the problem is no longer about eating. It becomes about overeating.

or less established, coping mechanisms have been taught and you are supposed to set your child on a voyage hoping she will reach the other side, that is, adulthood, intact. But this is not always the case. Peer influences are hard to resist, so no matter what kind of training you give them, you won't always be able to monitor what goes on outside your house. These influences are difficult to resist for you as an adult, so it is unrealistic to expect your child to achieve the impossible. This, of course, doesn't mean all your work has gone to naught, but it could mean your child's peers could trumpet the arrival of foods you didn't want them to eat. So what is it that you can do?

You keep it going. And then some.

In the war against unhealthy foods, this is the age group when you will realize there will be some battles you will not win.

Accept that it may not always go according to plan. Ultimately, there is a fine line between setting rules and controlling your child – one is enabling, the other disabling. But, as discussed earlier, you need to 'plough doggedly on' to keep ensuring that carefully formed habits do not, umm, deform. But what are the eating environments which little children have to face? Well, these are more insidious than you think and can sometimes creep up on your kids without you realizing it.

Nutritional Guidelines
Six to Nine Years

1. The Eating Environments

The Birthday Party

From what used to be a relatively tame affair consisting of four main things – a cake to cut, chips to eat, a hot samosa to gobble and a paper plate to eat it all out of – birthday parties have now become

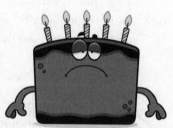

arenas of subtle or blatant one-upmanship. Now a child cannot progress to the next year without saying hello to their birthdays with a theme, a bouncy castle, a tattoo artist, a clown (no matter what the theme is, confusingly enough), an MC and a candy-floss machine. Of course, the details differ from party to party, but the fact is that many parents are pressured to host events which are sometimes on the scale of small weddings. While this is not a comment on excess, I am more concerned with what is served at these mega events. They sometimes include creamy cakes, fizzy drinks, pastries, chocolate fountains, carelessly strewn hard-boiled sweets, or even 'edible sweet decorations'. Because, you know, birthdays.

The Lunchbox

One of the most subtle proving-one's-worth grounds for a little child since school immemorial, the lunchbox is when all is revealed: how cool the child is based on what mummy/daddy/chief care provider 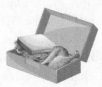 gives them to eat. Opening an awesome dabba unlocks the door to becoming a part of the 'it' crowd; food therefore becomes an important currency for surviving school. While it may not be as staunch as some of the other grounds for competition, like being a class topper/monitor or coming to school in a helicopter – I joke about the last one, but these days you never know – it can be one of the ways kids can pester you to include food in their daily diets that is not good for them.

The Play Date

While you can ignore the slightly frightening illustration – the children featured here seem to have very eerie smiles – the play date is a relatively newer kid on the block. It is usually where you get your 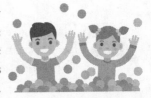 kids together with like-minded parents at homes, parks or activity centres, a date for both parent and child. But this is also where a perfectly well-behaved angel, spurred on by other not-so-perfectly-behaved angels, can suddenly morph into a red-faced sobbing mess because you didn't buy her the ice-cream sundae the other child's parents bought them, nutritional philosophies being different for different families.

The Bragging Rights

While all of the above can come under this title, this one especially refers to those marketing campaigns which target children. Whether it is chocolate eggs with toys in them – banned in 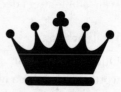 some countries – or collecting bottle caps of fizzy drinks for a chance to meet the captain of the Indian cricket team, sometimes food has literally nothing to do with food itself. It is, in fact, an entry point for something bigger, like the chance to be part of an exclusive club. And food is consumed for the most thoughtless reason of them all: as a stepping stone for a prize.

These environments could also be where eating can sometimes cross over to overeating, setting the stage for ignoring signals of satiety over time. The above list is by no means exhaustive, but highlighting them is more to establish the fact that:

 Children are exposed to environments where food has more to do with their own little place in life than as a source of nutrition.

And as it has been a while since we were children ourselves, it is hard to remember how crushing these small defeats can be in a child's world. Of course, I don't want to make the issue larger than it is because it is not always necessary that your child is affected by them – I have managed to keep my daughters' fingers out of many proverbial and literal pies (while my own fingers remain crossed). But I did want to emphasize nevertheless that staying healthy is as hard for children as it is for their parents, and it is the children I sometimes feel the most sympathy for.

What to Do When the School Feeds Your Child

Some preschools and schools have started the practice of providing lunches and sometimes even breakfasts to students. This ensures that even if you wanted to have a hand in creating daily meal plans for your children, your hands will be somewhat tied. You can get on board, however, by being an involved parent, to reassure yourself that both variety and nutrition is being represented in your child's daily diet.

II. The Coping Mechanisms

Feeling sorry for your children doesn't mean you have to give in. Dealing with life's little disappointments is part of life itself; you would be wise to carry on the good work by continuing to set an example as mentioned in great detail in the previous chapter (for those parents who have skipped straight to this part, it will give you the incentive to go back). But where the messages are concerned (what messages, you ask? Again, you will have to go back to the previous chapter. See, this is why you shouldn't skip to the good parts), they will have to be tailored to an older age group.

In addition to the tips given in the previous chapter, which are still relevant to the six to nine-ers – tweaked for an older child, of course – give them examples they can relate to. Explaining how the five fingers of nutrition will work for them using fairy tales may not work for a child who has crossed the fairy-tale age. For a more de-fairying approach, try relatable examples. Use logic instead of emotion. To that end, I have in my arsenal a trick I would like to share with you. It is called Mirror Mirror. Or Glass Class, if you fancy yourself a good rhyme.

This is where you gently drag your six to nine-year-old to make them stand in front of a mirror. Show them the benefit of healthy nutrition by pointing out to them how shiny their hair is because they have eaten their greens or how beautifully their skin glows because of all the Vitamin C they have consumed from the citrus family. I did that with my younger one, Amaira, and I swear it works. When they see the direct benefit of eating well on their own bodies, it gives them something to think about.

I would strongly advise you not to do the reverse, though. Dragging your child to a mirror to show her how pasty her skin has become and how straggly her hair is because she has been a bit too partial to all the sweeter things in life would not, in my opinion, be prudent. The broader point, of course, is to show your child the direct benefits of good nutrition and I would advise you to praise even minor changes. Mirror Mirror is a secular method – opening its arms to all kinds of foods – but you can alternatively choose various ways of conveying the benefits of more specific nutritional habits, like pointing out a good day in school because she drank lots of water or noting her handwriting looks good because she ate her breakfast.

Second, should your child show a propensity for liking all the 'wrong' things, you could give them one small 'cheat' a day (very limited quantities) where they can eat any one thing they like, no questions asked. You could designate this simply as snack time. This snack needs to be given on its own and not with the main meal, so as to encourage correct nutrient intake at mealtime and also to not spoil their appetite for healthier things. Case in point: one fine day my elder daughter, Ahaana, decided to push away her plate on account of feeling full. Respecting said choice, her plate was taken away and I thought she was about to leave the table to wash her hands. She stayed put and I, sensing something was definitely up, raised a curious eyebrow in her direction. She replied with both eyebrows raised, her big beautiful eyes open wide, and asked me for ice cream. 'I thought you were full,' I said to her, my eyebrow not backing down. 'I am, Mummy,' she smiled. 'My healthy food tummy is full. But my junk food stomach is empty.'

What a clever kid. I wonder where she gets it from.

Barring smart attempts to trick Mummy, I find this one special snack a day really works, though: children don't go crazy, they learn the value of portion control and even learn the value of food. This could also be modified to delay gratification: in case your child insists on having something that would be 'frowned upon' at home, you can always point them in the direction of an upcoming birthday party for them to satisfy their sweet tooth. Or teeth, if that is what you are dealing with.

Which kind of brings me to my third point. Don't divert from the plan in environments you can control. If you wish to establish a system of healthy eating plus a snack, stick to the plan and don't go off the beaten path. I believe that if you give in, Baby Blue/Black/Brown Eyes will begin to think that everything is negotiable and you will get far more resistance if you don't follow through with your intended promise. Needless to say, for the success of this plan, everyone from parents, grandparents, in-laws and your staff must speak the same language. Good luck telling your mother and your mother-in-law what to do with their grandchild, though. I will be here, safely sitting behind my laptop in a room far away from you.

III. The Nutritional Solutions

It seems more than a little ironic to me that so many foods targeted at little children are simply not good for them. So, when it comes to deciding what to prepare, do continue including all the five fingers of nutrition (elaborated on in the previous chapter) and make a fist even if your child may want to punch you with it. Portion sizes for this age group are still about two-thirds or more of the size of an adult's, so keep that in mind. Note that:

A five to six-year-old will eat about 60–70 per cent of what an adult does.

A child aged seven to nine will eat about 70–90 per cent of what an adult eats.

Estimate your servings accordingly.

Again, do treat the above portions as indicative and note that your child may feel more or less hungry from time to time, growth spurts being what they are. While you ensure that the five fingers of nutrition are properly represented in the daily food intake, here is some additional food for thought.

NO-SPILL-NO-LEAK TIFFINS

Non-Messy Foods for Six to Nine-Year-Olds

This is a three-week cyclical menu which ensures that the five fingers of nutrition are still making a fist. For ideas on making it more fun for your kids to eat, please refer to the Appendix.

TIFFIN IDEA 1

RICE, RAJMA AND VEGETABLES

- Carb: soft boiled rice
- Protein: rajma, more dense than watery
- Vitamins and minerals: dry bhindi or aloo in jeera
- Fats: as dictated by oil usage, and should be low oil. This will hold true for all other tiffin ideas

TIFFIN IDEA 2

FRANKIE WITH AVOCADO MASH

- Carb: roti
- Protein: avocado as the spread and grilled or boiled chicken or paneer with herbs
- Vitamins and minerals: carrot and cucumber added in

TIFFIN IDEA 3

HOMEMADE CORN TORTILLA CHIPS WITH SPINACH AND PANEER TOPPINGS

- Carb: tortilla chips (baked or fried). These can be made at home with makai atta and some oil, salt, pepper and herbs. Cut into easy-to-eat triangles
- Protein: paneer
- Vitamins and minerals: corn and spinach

TIFFIN IDEA 4

BAKED BEAN CANAPÉS WITH MIXED VEGETABLE CUTLET

- Carb: canapés made out of atta/roti, using a cupcake mould
- Protein: baked beans or homemade beans in tomato sauce
- Vitamins and minerals: mixed vegetable cutlet
- Pack the beans separately. It will be more fun for your child to assemble it herself, and munch along

TIFFIN IDEA 5

DAL PARATHA WITH SPINACH RAITA

- Carb: wheat/atta
- Protein: yellow moong dal and yogurt
- Vitamins and minerals: spinach

TIFFIN IDEA 6

HERBED CHICKEN OR SOYA WITH STEAMED RICE

- Carb: rice
- Protein: chicken or soyabean mince
- Vitamins and minerals: carrots and cucumbers

TIFFIN IDEA 7

YUMMY PASTA

- Carb: penne or fusilli
- Protein: chicken, paneer or cheese
- Vitamins and minerals: mushrooms, corn

TIFFIN IDEA 8

YIPPEE! NOODLES

- Carb: noodles
- Protein: egg
- Vitamins and minerals: spring onions, carrot, cabbage – all finely chopped

TIFFIN IDEA 9

NUTTY VEGETABLE PULAO

- Carb: rice
- Protein: soya chunks and nuts
- Vitamins and minerals: beans, carrots and potatoes

TIFFIN IDEA 10

VEGETABLE UPMA WITH PANEER CUTLET

- Carb: upma
- Protein: paneer cutlet
- Vitamins and minerals: carrots, beans and peas in the upma

TIFFIN IDEA 11

EGG FRANKIE WITH FRENCH FRIES OR SWEET POTATO WEDGES

- Carb: roti
- Protein: egg
- Vitamins and minerals: mushrooms and spinach

TIFFIN IDEA 12

CURD RICE WITH CRUNCHY BANANA CHIPS

- Carb: rice
- Protein: yogurt
- Vitamins and minerals: grated cucumber

TIFFIN IDEA 13

EGG SANDWICH WITH A SMALL BAR OF CHOCOLATE (Optional)

- Carb: bread
- Protein: boiled egg and cheese
- Vitamins and minerals: iceberg lettuce

TIFFIN IDEA 14

CHICKPEAS WITH METHI THEPLA

- Carbs: roti
- Protein: well-cooked chick peas
- Vitamins and minerals: methi

TIFFIN IDEA 15

OAT PANCAKES WITH HONEY AND BANANA SERVED WITH COLD MILK

- Carbs: oats
- Protein: milk in the pancake dough and served milk
- Vitamins and minerals: banana

Salt is to children what children are to white upholstery. It is not a good mix. Children must stay away from salty foods as much as possible, so takeaways, processed meats, salty biscuits, snacks, sauces and microwaveable ready-to-eat meals should all be taken off the table.

Water is the best drink known to man. Make it known to children. This refreshing, pure, healthy liquid is the best thirst quencher on the planet, out-quenching fruit juices, fruit drinks and energy drinks. Fruit drinks and juices are abundant in sugar, piling on way more than what your child needs. The best part about water is that it kills only thirst and not appetite, unlike the other drinks.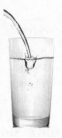

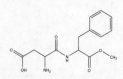 At no point should you give your children foods or beverages which contain artificial sweeteners. So sweetened drinks like diet colas, chewing gums or desserts which contain aspartame, saccharin or sucralose are a complete no-no. Sweeteners of this kind are just pure unadulterated chemicals made synthetically in a lab and have absolutely no nutritive value whatsoever. While aspartame is the absolute worst of the lot – it has been rejected by the American FDA a record eight times before it was included – and is associated with Alzheimer's Disease and cancer, among other not-so-cheerful side effects, the others have blood on their hands as well. Which is why even in my previous book, *Eat Delete*, I asked adults to give artificial sweeteners the boot. I would consider them to be one of the deadly sins of nutrition.

Also remember not to give six to nine-year-olds coffee, tea, colas, energy drinks or anything which contains caffeine. While caffeine is infamous for sleep disruption, tea also contains tannin, which messes with the little body's ability to absorb iron.

Cheese is actually a very convenient, whip-up-in-a-jiffy kind of food that can be a smart addition to lunch boxes, though it shouldn't be served every day since it is high in salt. Having said that, cottage cheese has 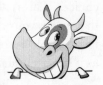 lower salt content than hard cheese. Other low-salt options include mozzarella, goat's cheese and cream cheese.

Breakfast is the most important meal of the day for any age group, and this especially holds true for the six to nine-ers and older because they have now graduated to the Big School, and have long days when they have to pay attention in class. Breakfast not only enables them to do that, it also helps control obesity and here is why: when you wake up after a night's sleep, your body has not had food for about eight to ten hours. The first meal you eat post that becomes breakfast because you are essentially 'break'ing the 'fast'. To that end, when you skip breakfast, your body thinks it is not receiving any food at all, and feels it is being starved. It then stores the next meal it gets as fat as a way to create a future energy reserve because it doesn't know when it will get food next. Skipping breakfast promotes fat storage. Egg, milk and toast, for example, would be a complete breakfast or any meal, for that matter, which has a healthy carb, good protein and/or milk.

I wanted to leave you with one last thought. While the focus of the chapter is how to handle a child's response to different eating environments, I wish to point out that the six to nine age group is also the phase when picky eating ends and the curious phase starts. Which means that it is not always a steady stream of competitiveness or feeling-out-of-place-ness which guides your child towards making unorthodox food choices. This is also a time of genuine self-propelled interest that makes your child reach out for things not always good for her. I would recommend that you pick your battles because, as it has been said once, you can't win them all.

THE ABCs OF OLDER CHILDHOOD NUTRITION: SIX TO NINE YEARS

Chapter Summary

 In the six to nine age group, while both the parent and child still have nutritional responsibilities, there is a new fix in the mix: peers. Their influence could trumpet the entry of foods you had no intention of bringing to the table.

 Your child could be exposed to eating environments more influential than you think. These could include birthday parties, lunch boxes, play dates and more.

 Sometimes your child winds up eating junk or processed food for reasons which have nothing to do with the food itself.

 Keep setting an example for children of these ages too. Make mealtime a priority, encourage healthy experimentation, engage your child in conversation, take their help in preparing meals, share new foods and keep the meal environment happy and positive. However, tweak your messages for an older audience, when needed.

 Use logic instead of emotion with older children. Show the direct results of good nutrition by showing her how it reflects in her hair, skin and performance at school.

 You could also allow her one special snack a day. If she is overweight, it should be given once or twice a week so your child doesn't feel too deprived.

Don't divert from the plan in environments you can control. Ensure adherence to mealtimes and special snacks; try not to bend, no matter what the circumstance. If you start relaxing your own rules, your child may think everything else is negotiable too. The best way to ensure this is to get the cooperation of everyone else in the house, like your spouse, staff or your child's grandparents.

 Please be careful of too much salt, sugar and processed foods. Ideally, the latter shouldn't feature in your child's diet at all.

 Water is the best drink known to man. Make it known to children. Anything else either has too much sugar or is simply not good for your child.

 Teas, coffees, colas and caffeinated drinks are a no-no at this age. Caffeine interferes with sleep and tannin interferes with iron absorption.

 Never give your child anything that contains artificial sweeteners like aspartame, sucralose and saccharine. I cannot emphasize this enough.

 Ultimately, realize that there are some battles you may not win when peers and the environment start to influence your children nutritionally. And while this may not be a given, keep focusing on the road ahead and continue to teach your child nutritional responsibility.

Hansel and Gretel

Pester Power and Nutrition

Hansel and Gretel was published in the early 1800s, but it is incredible how relevant the story of the wicked witch luring innocent children to eat a house made of sweets is even two centuries later. The witch may have morphed into a faceless company and the sweets may have turned into compounds like high fructose corn syrup, but what hasn't changed is the luring of children who are far too young to know better. If adults cannot resist the psychological tactics used to get people to buy things, then how much of a fight can defenceless little children put up?

Like it or not, advertisements targeted at children are here to stay. Brands will try their hardest to sell to a target that is easily distracted by shiny things, cartoon characters, on-ground events, free toys as well as online and TV ad bombardment. In a study that was conducted in India[1] among three to twelve-year-old children and their parents, it was found that an eye-bulging, mind-boggling 82 per cent of children were influenced by in-store ads of chocolates and biscuits. In the same study, a massive 73 per cent of children surveyed were likely to buy a confectionary product because a celebrity or cartoon character is associated with it.[2] In other words, Hansel and Gretel are being lured all the time. Not realizing that they are.

There is also a term given to buying decisions made by parents buckling under relentless demand from their children. It is called pester power or the power-to-drive-your-parents-crazy-as-you-roll-on-the-floor-of-the-supermarket-crying-until-they-give-in-and-buy-you-what-you-want. I am not going into too much detail about many of the processed foods which have these 'sweet deals', because the fact that there is very little nutritive value to these foods has been established. What is of greater concern to me is that the same study suggested that 77 per cent of parents agreed to buy their child whatever she wanted when she insisted. Which means that I would like to help you with any tool you may need when your child insists you buy them. The food, not the tools. If she is going to spend the bulk of her time while you shop for groceries writhing on the floor next to the chocolates section, bawling her eyes out, you may as well have some strategies in place to say 'No'.

What works for me is a balloon-pop strategy in which I burst the balloon or the aura surrounding the food in question. I have always told my kids that foods which are so heavily advertised are those that supermarkets cannot sell, either because they cause problems in the long-term or just the fact that nobody likes them. In other words, they cannot sell because they are no good. You can use other approaches depending on your child's personality, like maybe telling them a particular sweet makes their tongue go purple, which may leave a permanent stain over time. Barring a few hiccups, this has worked so far and they now ask me to buy things after giving a little more thought to it.

What has also been successful as a strategy is if I reduce exposure to the medium and cut off ads at the source.

Limiting TV and iPad time is what I am extremely strict about, and not just from a nutritional perspective. Even between these two, I prefer the iPad for my daughters because they can play games versus watching shows or cartoons with irresistible protagonists who compel them to make almost irresistible pitches for foods I am very much resistant to buy.

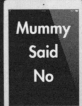

 Of course, the only way to not give in is, quite simply, to not give in.

Never give in when they are pleading, crying, throwing tantrums or giving you the silent treatment because they believe that so long as they keep at it, you will relent. No matter how tempting the prospect of throwing in the towel, the 'I-said-no-don't-ask-me-again' tactic will make them give up after sometime if they realize you are serious. Just hang in there. It will pass.

From a broader, more legislative perspective, banning junk food ads may not have an immediate impact on the reduction of childhood obesity rates because the problem of obesity is usually more complex and cannot be attributed to only one direct source. However, even though these kinds of moves would probably have a more long-term indirect impact, going from the data it is clear that marketing is definitely exacerbating the problem and not mitigating it. I feel that if ads or marketing strategies which are specifically targeted towards children are banned, parents would sit up and take more notice because of the overall seriousness a ban adds. It would also allow the government to take things a little more seriously and, you never know, maybe make junk food part of a public healthcare initiative like the polio or 'Clean India' campaigns. For nutritionists whose job it is to suggest healthy solutions, it is with dismay that we see the introduction of so many foods which rank so poorly on health indexes and contain so many chemicals which seem to find favour with many children. These foods should never be part of any child's digestive system. At this moment, though, the seriousness of the message is not being conveyed and there is some sort of eerie status quo which somehow suggests that many of these foods are nutritionally acceptable. When, in fact, they are not.

There is a growing movement, though, where children are being urged to use pester power for something more positive: using their considerable influence to pester their parents to do more for the environment. If schools influence their kids who can then influence their parents to take action for climate change, it can propel the world in a whole new direction. Pester power is not always a bad thing.[2]

Whatever you do, please keep in mind that while you are putting up resistance against their demands when they are being unreasonable, they are just little children who are being led astray by some bright blinking lights. They don't know any better.

But you do.

The End

Goldilocks and the Three Bears

Constructing a Healthy Nutritional Environment

When Goldilocks walked into an empty house, everything was laid out for her: bed, porridge, all within easy reach. Tempted by so many things on offer, she ate someone else's porridge, broke someone else's furniture and slept on someone else's bed, only to be rudely awakened by the original tenants, the Three Bears. While the moral of this story is that you need to lock your door especially if you're living in an isolated area, the other takeout from this tale is that if something is easy to access, it's difficult to resist. If it's lying around, it's harder to ignore.

If your cupboards are groaning with high-calorie goodies or your shelves are weighed down by all the stuff most nutritionists will tell you to run away from, you cannot expect a child *not* to be swayed by the lure of all things sugary or fatty. Will power, in essence, is a more adult concept and it is something most adults themselves are struggling with, so expecting a child to be very disciplined all the time is to expect a bit much. A child's eating environment at home is an extremely common way to inculcate *unhealthy* eating habits in your little one, so if you want your child to stick to a nobler nutritional path, you would have to ask them not to do as you say, but do as you chew. To that end, you will have to:

Stock

Eating healthy starts with access to health. If your fridge is brimming with the goodness of fresh vegetables or if your fruit bowls actually contain fruit, and not car keys and old receipts, then you have already created an environment that promotes healthy eating. Variety is the spice of life and this also holds true for stocking. Raw ingredients are rarely fattening, so from fresh and dry fruits to fresh veggies of so many kinds, to eggs, grains, lean meats and low-fat dairy, there are so many healthy routes to delicious eating. Pre-prepare snacks like homemade hummus/hung curd sandwich spreads or baked snacks or even homemade frozen yogurt (just blend fruit with low-fat yoghurt and freeze for a few hours) and you have some ready solutions when your children are feeling peckish.

Sacrifice

Unhealthy foods should be banished from sight: children cannot ask for what they do not see. If you really must eat junk, I would suggest you lock it up in the same place you put your wedding jewellery or your passport, and only bring it out when the kids have gone to bed or for art class. If Mummy or Daddy needs a restorative that isn't alcoholic, make sure that your children are not there to see you eat it. Having said that, it will really be to your benefit to junk the junk food. But this is a book for children.

Slow

Limit access to media/TV shows because, as we all know, advertisements are a trigger for junk food. Put yourself in the tiny little shoes of your children. As a kid, would you be able to resist images of chocolate oozing out of doughnuts? Or the shiny toy that comes free with the value meal? The less your kids see, the less they remember, the less they pester, the more you relax. Having said that, this is way easier said than done, and the last thing I want to do is preach when I sometimes struggle to do this myself. Do what you can do. But don't forget to keep trying.

Share

While this has already been mentioned before, set an example at the table. If you are dreaming of a day when your child would crave cucumber sticks, you would have to be the one who not only introduces them but appears to like them. Make a happy face, go 'Mmmmm', say 'Yummy in your tummy', and watch your slightly bewildered child pick up the same and follow suit. Happy associations with healthy food go a long way in establishing a good relationship with them.

Out of all the environments that your child will be exposed to, the home is the easiest to control, but for complete success, everyone needs to pitch in, from family members to staff. And while it may seem difficult initially, the entire family – and not just the children – will benefit as they get reacquainted with the best that food has to offer.

The End

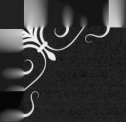
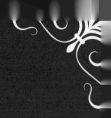

The Three Little Pigs

And the Big Bad Wolves of Nutrition

If you are a stickler for detail, no, there aren't any pigs in this particular piece but I really wanted to use the phrase 'Big Bad Wolf' and this is the only way I could do it. There may not be pigs here but fact is that there *are* bad wolves in the nutritional ecosystem and these aren't ingredients or recipes but are, quite simply, relationships. Relationships with food.

In my previous book, *Eat Delete*, I had outlined some key relationships with food that most of us have whether we realize it or not, some of which can be detrimental to long-term health. While some of these have been unwittingly imparted to us by our parents and some have been picked up over time, you may find yourself nodding at some because this is what you were taught as a child yourself. I have reproduced some of the following from the perspective of child nutrition:

Food As Reward

Did Agastya do his homework? Did Vedica finish her palak ki sabzi? Food as reward can be a key way of disciplining children, and what makes it such a popular relationship with food is that it works so well. What this tends to do, as mentioned in this book, is that it tends to pit one food (dessert/sweets) against another not-so-cool food, amplifying its perceived value. The reward foods then become 'forbidden', making them all the more appealing. Food rewards will typically be foods that are sugary, fatty, highly calorific and dubiously nutritive. And bribing with food – whether it is rewarding yourself or your child – could be a habit that could last a lifetime.

Food As Comfort

Cooking a special meal when your child has the sniffles is different from feeding a child his favourite food when he has broken his favourite toy. Emotional feeding and emotional eating could be a disruptive coping mechanism, as is teaching a child that the solution to any problem lies at the bottom of a tub of ice cream or in the depths of a fridge. There are many other coping mechanisms for life's disappointments, which include dance, exercise, talking, playing outdoors, therapy, colouring, or any other hobby that your child likes. Can he be taught to seek solace in something other than a plate?

Food As Enemy

This is especially true for older children, in their pre-teens and teens. Physical appearance becomes a key social barometer during puberty and suddenly good, healthy food groups like carbs become the enemy, depriving your child of nutrition at the time he needs it the most. Boys want to typically get bigger and stronger, eschewing balanced meals for high-protein diets. Girls usually want to get thinner and 'smaller', pushing away large chunks of food or nixing food groups like carbs altogether or not drinking water because, like water in a balloon, they mistakenly believe it increases their size. The phase of adolescence could also be where many eating disorders, unfortunately, come into their own.

 We have all experienced, taught and passed on some of these relationships and it is a cycle we sometimes perpetuate without realizing.

Prima facie, these big bad wolves seem like a forgone conclusion – with the exception of maybe the last – and I don't want to sound judgemental or impractical if you are seeing yourself in these pages.

What we must also realize as grown-ups is that no relationship is perfect and these include relationships with food, which are very hard to extricate ourselves from. Highlighting these then becomes a matter of engendering consciousness. So that we become aware of our behaviour as parents. So that we minimize using food as a weapon. So that everybody wins.

The End

Pre-teen and Teen Nutrition
Age Ten to Fifteen Years

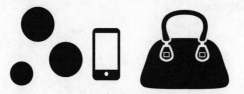

Comparative sizes of a child's stomach between ten and fifteen
years. Indicative. All bets are off.

The pre-teen and teen years can safely be defined as the 'wonder years'. Where you wonder what happened to your formerly obedient, hugging, kissing, agreeable child who did mostly whatever you asked them to. Where you wonder whether you were this kind of teenager to your parents. Whether you need to call them right now to ask, just to feel better. And if you will ever get through this spurt of growth, and what lies on the other side. I can tell you that since we all made it through puberty and most of us are still speaking to our parents – and listening to them, whether we like it or not – this phase with your child will pass. Wonder no more.

But yes, nutritional guidance at this stage in your child's life is easy to give and very hard to implement. You are not just dealing with influences of peers, ads, social media, but your parenting is now going head-to-head with a surge of hormones. Your child is growing up and with it will come a reminder that so are you. Features are becoming more defined, clothes are being grown out of, the self-consciousness of appearance is starting to rear its head, a head that spends a lot more time in front of the mirror. But they are still not all that grown-up, so it doesn't mean that the old rules don't apply anymore. They are still somewhere between ten to fifteen years old and even if they are on the cusp of adulthood, it doesn't mean they don't need good nutrition. In fact, they need it more than ever.

Nutritional Guidelines

Ten to Fifteen Years

I. The Last Big Growth Spurt

To quote the very first line of a study published in the *Indian Journal of Endocrinology and Metabolism*, 'Nutrition is one of the most important factors affecting pubertal development.'[1] Fairly straightforward, one might say. You need food to grow and boy, growth does happen at this stage:[2]

1.   Height – or linear growth – increases greatly during this thunderous time at the rate of approximately 5 cm/year in pre-pubertal kids, 8.3 cm/year in pubertal girls and 9.5 cm/year in pubertal boys. That is a lot of growth right there.

2.   Height will continue to 'spurt' for anywhere between two to three years, hitting the end of the road for girls at the age of sixteen-and-a-half years and about seventeen to eighteen[3] for boys. This is Stage Five of development when a teen starts to look like an adult physically. Adults are Stage Five for the rest of their life. However, there may be a small increase in height after the age of nineteen years for girls.

3.   About *half* the ideal adult body weight is gained during
      the teen years, after the age of fourteen.

4.   Weight increases at the rate of 9 kilos *per year* for boys
      and 8.3 kilos for girls. The weight gain in males consists
      almost entirely of lean tissue.

5.   You would think that the age of ten was far too tender to
      hit puberty, but the truth is that most girls enter puberty
      from the age of eight till they are thirteen. For boys, it is
      a bit later; from ten till the age of fifteen.[4]

Healthy food is needed now, more than ever. And a
surprising amount of it too.

Fix your eyes on these numbers:

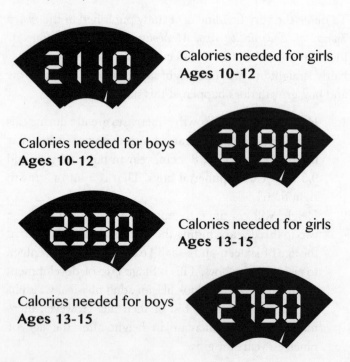

2110 Calories needed for girls
Ages 10-12

Calories needed for boys
Ages 10-12 2190

2330 Calories needed for girls
Ages 13-15

Calories needed for boys
Ages 13-15 2750

This data comes to you straight from the Indian Council of Medical Research, so this is an Indian recommended dietary allowance.[5]

 These calorie counts are more than what most adults need; that is how important nutrition is at the puberty stage.

The last time growth and development was this rapid was when the now pre-teen or teen was a tiny baby. As they are both growth spurts, infancy and adolescence are when nutrition and healthy food are needed more than ever. But the question is, are they getting enough?

The answer, I am afraid, is no.

II. The Teen Eating Environment

When your teen or pre-teen is burying his head into his cell phone (presumably he will start to nag you for one when he has crossed the age of ten or eleven), chances are he is usually not discussing his homework assignments of the day. He is testing the waters, even if he is not drinking enough of it. With independence comes the ability to explore nutritional choices of his own. And all of them are not necessarily good ones. His eating environment could be summed up in the following texts:

Hello, light of my life. I've made your favourite anda curry and pulao for your dabba. Please eat everything. Big kissy.

Ma, please stop calling me that. It's embarrassing. And I'm too old for kisses.

While the answer usually has no resemblance to the question, you have to deduce from the subtext of the text in such situations. You will find out the answer only once the lunch has come back from school, sometimes eaten but more often half-eaten, a thanda response to the anda. Whether in school or after school, teens are more likely to eat away from home – even if home has been delivered to them – and supervision is not always possible unless you have hired detectives. For which I laud you for your commitment.

> Hello, blot on the landscape. Are you home at four?

> Out.

Since you are not allowed to call him the light of your life, by replacing it with the 'blot on the landscape' line (thank you, again, Wodehouse), do not expect your child to necessarily get the joke. You may receive a clear and succinct answer to the question, though. Indeed, you should thank your stars if you get any answer at all. Teens are more likely to go to fast-food outlets to 'hang' after school activities, so they do have exposure to undesirable foods, to put it mildly.

> Morning, Your Royal Highness. I have packed your favourite cheese sandwich with the sides cut off. Lots of love, your namma.

> Aw, Ma. I don't eat those anymore. Love you.

Teens' tastes change when they hit puberty along with changes of mood, and they show a marked preference for fat if they are not watching their weight. Boys also show more love for protein, probably due to their belief that it builds muscle. On the other hand, girls are more likely to crave sweets because of a rise in their oestrogen levels. Excess fat and sweets are especially areas of concern at this stage because of their propensity to tip the weighing scales to the other side.

Please finish your food, love. Your dabbas keep coming back.

?!

Teenagers are fairly resistant to being told what to do, especially what, where and how to eat, even though they need more protein, calcium, iron, folate and zinc than before. But we now know that improper nutrition at this crucial development stage can affect what is called The Three As: Academics, Athletics and Attitude.

III. The Five Fingers of Nutrition for Ten to Fifteen-Year-Olds

Given the tone of the previous text messages, the tendency of your no-longer-a-baby baby to be undernourished or malnourished is far greater, even though he seems to eat all the time, because he is not getting the right foods. Girls who are menstruating are at further risk of iron deficiency. It also doesn't help that the inability to get enough calcium or protein during this time may lead to the damage of bone or muscle growth. But enough doom and gloom. Let's talk solutions. Here is what the five fingers of nutrition look like for your ten to fifteen-year-old.

VITAMINS

In puberty, both boys and girls need 20-30 per cent more vitamin intake. And even though it is best to get these from food, erratic eating habits could mean vitamin deprivation, so supplements may be the best medium for these nutrients to enter the body. Do check with your doctor first, though.

MINERALS

Twenty per cent more **IRON** is needed by boys for muscle growth while 33 per cent more for menstruating girls. Indian Recommended Daily Allowance (RDA) states: boys (ten to twelve) = 21 mg and 32 mg (thirteen to fifteen) while girls (ten to twelve) = 27 mg, which is the same for thirteen to fifteen years. When it comes to **ZINC**, teen boys need 33 per cent more while girls need about 20 per cent more than before. **Indian RDA** for both sexes is 9 mg for ten to twelve years and 11 mg for thirteen to fifteen years. As for **CALCIUM,** both teen boys and girls need about 33 per cent more (1200 mg as opposed to 800 mg as required earlier).

FLUIDS

I cannot lay enough stress on the importance of good old water at this stage. Colas, fruit drinks, energy drinks and anything which is processed and comes out of a bottle, packet or a can that is not simple plain water is a pointless addition to your pre-teen and teen diet. No less than ten to twelve glasses a day for your child, more if he is the sporty, outdoorsy, athletic type.

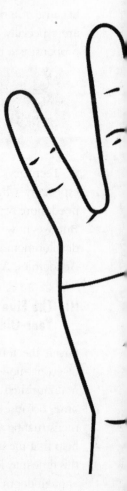

FATS

It is important to make a distinction between bad fats and smart fats. The brain may be developed by this age, but it is still creating connections, making this another spurt of growth for the brain. At precisely the time they need it the most, teens tend to let go of good fats – essential fatty acids, either to compete in athletics or to start the process of looking fit and attractive – or add more bad fats, including more saturated and hydrogenated kinds, in their food. The only problem with cutting out fat is that the good fats tend to get the boot as well. Teen brains need more fish and nuts, and less fries.

PROTEIN

Boys need about 25 per cent more protein or about 0.5 g more per pound of body weight, or about 15 more grams daily than a pre-teen. Teen girls need less protein than boys. Indian RDA for boys (10-12 y) = 40 g and 55 g (13-15 y) while girls (10-12) = 40 g and 52 g (13-15 y). Choose good lean protein like low-fat milk, low-fat cheese, curds, paneer, chicken, soyabean, eggs, fish, dal.

CARBS

Your pre-teen and teen should make good friends with good carbs like whole wheat, corn, rice, ragi, oats and also bread, noodles or pasta, in controlled portions.

The sources of these foods have been mentioned in previous chapters but I am including sample diets which would best help balance them out. Please refer to the Appendix for the following:

Of course, there is many a slip betwixt the cup and the lip; you can take a horse to water but you can't make it drink ten to twelve glasses a day. How can we best motivate our children to best eat their daily bread? Well, you can tweak the tips I have elaborated in the earlier chapters, but here is what you can bring to the table for the ten to fifteen-year-old. And even older, for that matter.

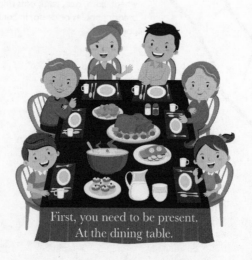

First, you need to be present. At the dining table.

While this may not apply to the ten to twelve-year-olds, as your child grows, he may not always want to eat with the family at the dinner table, with homework, TV, screentime or texting being what it is. Puberty is a time for privacy and they may just prefer to explore their new worlds alone. It is even more important therefore to insist that mealtimes are sacred and eating with the family is non-negotiable. You can use this time to be a gentle support as he goes through this very difficult and sometimes confidence-denting time, as mealtimes are a good time to communicate. And while communicating, maybe you can also:

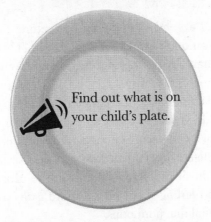

Find out what is on your child's plate.

Apart from finding out what is going on in your child's life by asking him direct questions, mealtimes are a great source of non-verbal communication. It is when you observe both what your child is eating and what is eating him. It is a great place to pick up cues which he may not otherwise directly express – not because he doesn't want to but because he may not be aware of what is going on himself. Is he trying to build his body by reaching for a second helping of chicken? Is she trying to lose weight by not reaching out for much at all?

You can understand a lot of what is going on nutritionally, psychologically and physiologically by just adhering to a simple breakfast, lunch and dinner schedule.

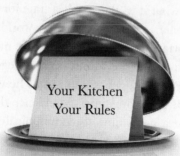

Your Kitchen
Your Rules

Try to set a good example by not getting food into the house that you don't want your child to eat. This may mean you might have to be the sacrificial lamb yourself by not eating the processed foods you dream of when you sleep. Like we had spoken about in the chapter on nutrition for six to nine-year-olds, you need to set an example. 'Do as I say, not as I do' is not a convincing enough argument for the curious, logical, intelligent millennial. You can also set a nutritious example by involving your children in the process of food shopping and letting them play a more active role in their own nutritional magnum opus.

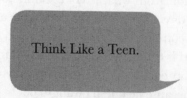

Think Like a Teen.

What do teenagers want in the end? The boys may want to grow taller, the girls may feel left out if they don't get training bras, and both may want to clear their skin. Hey presto! Here is where you swoop in with what nutrition can do to help them achieve their goals. Here is where you bung in all the WCS (worst case scenarios, for the uninitiated) of carbonated beverages, sweeteners and processed foods. Tell them how sugary foods spike their blood-sugar levels only to send them crashing down again, making them feel tired, lethargic and low. Tell them how overeating – especially the wrong foods – could render their afternoon study sessions totally unproductive and get in the way of what they want to achieve. Tell them how cutting out fat and starving themselves could not only affect their bodies but also their brains. See what your child seems to want the most – whether it is their growth, their appearance, their emotional stability, their academic performance or making it into the football team. There is always a nutritional lesson embedded in all of these things.

IV. Eating for the Three As: Athletics, Academics and Attitude

Nutrition for Athletics

Whether or not you had a sporty gene, it is always lovely to see your kid leap over hurdles on the obstacle course like a gazelle while you trip on carpets, unlike one. Sports nutrition is a special breed of eating and does require the person to eat as per his level of activity. What your child is doing with the expensive shoes he made you buy qualifies as sport if it involves one-and-a-half to two hours of activity at a time; he will need to eat more to keep up with the energy these activities demand. More training means more food, both in quality and quantity, so here is what I would recommend for your budding Olympian:

CALCIUM Calcium is crucial to the development of strong bones and the prevention of stress fractures, both important for the athlete. Foods that are calcium rich include low-fat dairy like yogurt, milk and cheese. Other sources include members of the leafy green family like spinach, kale, turnips, bhindi and pak choi.

PROTEIN We know, of course, that protein is an essential building block, helping in the building and repairing of muscles. Addition of protein will help repair muscular wear and tear. Protein also helps with muscle recovery as it leads to reduced muscle soreness the day after heavy physical activity. While protein-rich foods include eggs, lean meats, fish, dairy products, dals, nuts and soy, vegetarians usually find it a bit harder to get good protein from plant sources. For them, I'd recommend quinoa or soyabean, both of which are 100 per cent reference proteins (all of the protein content of the food is absorbed by the body), and are very versatile foods.

IRON Iron is the messenger that carries oxygen to all the parts of the human body. A deficiency thereof could lead to your child feeling tired more easily, clearly counterproductive to the whole sports thing. Girls who are both menstruating and athletic have a bit of a double whammy as they could lose some iron every month during their periods. Keep up the iron-rich diet by including more lean meats (chicken, tuna), eggs, leafy green vegetables, dry fruits and fortified wholegrains.

CARBS Very important to the training process, carbs are a vital source of fuel for the sportsperson. Carb loading – a practice where athletes eat lots of carbs prior to the game/event as a source of energy – is prevalent but should be done with caution. Healthy carb sources include bread, dosa, idli, rice, wheat, dalia and poha.

Meals of Champions

Suggestions for snacks and meals even during the sports off-season include:

1. Low-fat yogurt with granola. Throw in a banana for good measure.

2. Egg sandwich.

3. Frankie.

4. Poha with sprouts.

5. Oats porridge and almonds.

6. Any traditional meal that consists of roti, vegetables and dal.

7. Chicken or vegetable sandwich and fruit for lunch.

8. For dinner, grilled chicken/paneer with steamed rice and vegetables or pasta with red sauce, along with a salad.

9. Snacks could include khakra, nuts, dried fruits, crackers, idli, dosa or fruit.

I also wanted to point out that various coaches and trainers have their own nutritional philosophies about what a student should eat and drink for peak athletic performance. While they are experienced and may be well-meaning, it is better to receive the final go-ahead from your doctor or nutritionist based on your child's health report and vitamin and mineral levels. It is unlikely that any sweeping nutritional prescription will work for every child, so it is best to check in with people who have access to more information and can help you and your child make that decision.

Sports can take the juice out of you, quite literally, as it can dehydrate you like few things can. Physical activity can zap energy, strength, bring heat-exhaustion related illnesses with it and even the mildest dehydration can affect performance. A sporty kid knows that it is important to top up on fluids but does he know that water is the best fluid of them all? Although there are tonnes of sports drinks available on a supermarket shelf near you, water will do the trick just as well, thank you. Also note that thirst is not a reliable symptom of dehydration – your child may be dehydrated but not feel thirsty at all – so 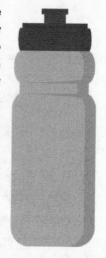 encourage him to top up on fluids before the activity and at fifteen to twenty-minute intervals during it. Drink afterwards as well to restore what has been lost as sweat.

Second, sometimes there is also pressure exerted – either implicitly or explicitly – about slimming down or bulking up to enhance athletic performance. Please ensure that your child does not employ any starvation tactics or other nutritional shortcuts to reach his goals, no matter how balefully he looks up at you at the dining table. Any transformative effort must be complemented by a goody-two-shoes healthy diet and exercise routine. There is no other scientifically proven way to change a child's physiology without damaging it.

Game Day Nutrition

How to prep your sportstar on the day of an event:

1. A high-carb, moderate protein, low-fat meal two hours before the activity. High-fat and high-fibre foods take longer to digest and can upset the stomach.

2. A lighter meal or snack if your child is eating less than two hours before the game. This could be easily digestible carbohydrates like fruit, bread or biscuits.

3. Feed them carbohydrates thirty minutes before a high intensity event and then again two hours post the event, because your child's body is rebuilding muscle tissue and restoring energy and fluids up until twenty-four hours post the activity. It is better to replenish with healthy proteins, fats and carbs rather than unhealthy snacks.

4. Don't forget to pack lots of water.

Nutrition for Academics

I remember once one of my more jet-setting clients walking into my consulting room, mourning the loss of her annual December vacation. I looked up, surprised, expecting to be regaled by a fancy-pants itinerary. But, alas, forget fancy, there were no pants this year either. The annual vacation had been postponed on account of exams, she said. She looked a bit mature, shall we say, to be sitting for exams, but then she thought to clarify. 'My son's exams, Pooja. Tenth. Boards.'

In today's millennial parenting scenario, the whole family has to prepare for the exam when the child takes it. A far cry from the days where your far cries were rarely heard by parents, whose job during an undeniably difficult and stressful time was to make sure you were fed and ensure that you reached the examination hall on time. As is often seen, there is a tendency during exams for students to lean towards comfort food like processed, fattening and sugary junk. While this may definitely provide some psychological reprieve, it may not satisfy the purpose of the exam itself. Richer, heavier foods are more difficult to digest and divert blood from the brain and reroute it to the digestive system. Blood brings oxygen to the brain and diverting it means that the brain won't work as well as it should. While you basically do need to ensure your child eats a balanced meal and sleeps well, you can bump up the following foods:

Protein

Protein helps with both the retention of information as well as the recall of it. Good-quality lean protein like dal, eggs, fish, chicken, soyabean and quinoa work well. Eggs have something called choline, which aids both memory and cognition.

Water

Dehydration could cause headaches and tiredness – not the best formula for remembering formulae. About two litres of water a day should help keep your child hydrated. Also, since the hunger and thirst centres in the brain are set so close together, the brain becomes confused and sometimes pushes the child to eat when they are merely *thirsty*. To prevent overeating, keep him drinking adequate water.

Good Fats

While I have mentioned this in the protein aisle, fish is also a tremendous source of good omega-3 fats, which help with the working of the brain. Vegetarians can opt for chia seeds, flaxseeds or walnuts, all of which are great sources of omega-3.

Fresh Vegetables and Fruits

These are great for building immunity. The last thing your child needs is to fall sick during exams.

Pumpkin Seeds

This is a great source of zinc which, in turn, is a great way to boost both memory and thinking. Pumpkin also has magnesium, Vitamin B and tryptophan, all of which help keep your child's mood up and ensure deep sleep.

Warm Milk and Herbal Teas

These help induce both sleep and calm.

A Carb Snack an Hour Before Bedtime

This will ease the path of sleep-promoting amino acids to the brain.

Caffeine

As both childhood and adolescence are phases of growth and brain development, anything that interferes with sleep is a bad idea. Enter caffeine – classified as a drug that stimulates the central nervous system – with its ability to disrupt sleep, hamper nutrition, enhance obesity and kick-start dental problems. Put that together with a growing child and you have got more problems than you can deal with. And it is not just about the side effects, but about caffeine's potential ability to influence a preference for drinks and sweets. To add to this, there is also evidence – albeit from animal studies – that caffeine influences the brain to increase its response to (prohibited) drugs. Yikes.

Unlike its common association with coffee, caffeine is found in tea, energy drinks (that sometimes contain up to five times the caffeine level as compared to coffee, and are advertised to teens) and, surprisingly, in something as seemingly decaffeinated as chocolate. A 30-g slab of chocolate could contain almost as much caffeine as a cup of decaffeinated coffee. Dark chocolate and hot chocolate also have caffeine. The only thing that doesn't have caffeine is white chocolate.

Caffeine can cause the following problems in your children:

1. Headaches

2. Stomach issues

3. Nervousness and jumpiness

4. Problems with concentration

5. Problems with sleeping

6. Elevated heart rate and blood pressure

And even very little intake of it can cause these symptoms in children.

Nutrition for Attitude

You know your child's face anywhere. Or, rather, you know your child's *faces* anywhere. His many moods have been etched into your heart and you recall them, sometimes with fondness and sometimes with not so much fondness. Fond or not, your child has his phases like any human being. But if you do see a decidedly long period of grump and slump, could it be the food he is eating? In 'Nutrition for Attitude',

I will briefly touch upon those foods which could be causing your Gus to become gloomy.

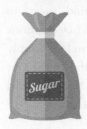

It is a well-established fact that sugar is a maverick pilot, making you soar and then sending you crashing down to earth even before the seatbelt sign has come on. Sugary foods are notorious for providing a quick burst of energy, but making you feel more tired, sluggish and grumpy in the end. Savoury processed foods could also have as much sugar as their more insidious sugary bedfellows. A diet which is high in sugary/processed foods has been associated with depression, sleep issues and cognitive delay.[6] Doesn't look so sweet after all.

MSG or Monosodium Glutamate is a flavour enhancer used mainly in Chinese cooking – although keep a lookout for it in other cuisines. It is guilty of causing changes in mood and behaviour. Other preservatives include anything in the nitrate or nitrite family as well as sodium benzoate, which I must add is found in juices targeted to children.

Artificial colouring is another red flag that causes kids to see, umm, red. Often tucked away in relatively innocuous foods like bread and dairy products, this particular substance causes anxiety, headaches and mood swings in children. Stay as far away as you can from products which are 'coloured' with Yellow No. 5, Red No. 40 and Blue No. 1. Products containing artificial colouring have been banned in most countries. It is now your turn to ban it too.

The last on the hit list is allergens. When a child is allergic or intolerant of certain foods like nuts, dairy, corn, soy and eggs, it does bring about changes in his behaviour. So it is best to rule out any problem regarding allergies with the help of a qualified professional to check if the cause is nutritional.

Before you brand your ward a problem child (owing to his mood swings), put on your deerstalker hat like Sherlock Holmes did and become a detective. He could, in fact, simply be in nutritional distress. And while unhealthy foods can wreak havoc on a child's physiological and psychological make-up, the resulting tsunami of chemicals can be a very curable imbalance.

V. Nutrition and Body Image

If I had a penny for every time someone came into my clinic with an exaggerated negative body image, I would have single-handedly ended world hunger by now. This is probably the downside of the work I do; I see someone putting so much pressure on themselves to lose a few kilos that I don't know if losing the extra weight will make any difference to the way they feel about themselves. My heretofore joke book will take a break during this discussion of the sad flipside of nutrition: the eating disorder.

Adolescence – and the onset of it – is a difficult time for a parent, but more so for teenagers. It is heartbreaking to note that the average age for the onset of eating disorders like Anorexia Nervosa and Bulimia Nervosa is during the teen years, and the struggle with it can take years to overcome. Although an eating disorder is a child of many parents and can be attributed to environmental, psychological, biological and personal causes, the fact is that teenagers are highly at risk.

While they are slamming doors and spending a lot of time in their rooms, teens are also experiencing a period of such stress, confusion and anxiety that it can make them do things out of character just to fit in. The self-consciousness that accompanies physical transformation and pre-pubescent/pubescent awkwardness along with romantic and sexual feelings lead them to grapple with self-esteem issues they have probably never had before, at least on this scale. Hormones can have mental, physical, psychological and emotional repercussions on teens. Trying to cement their place in the world can be difficult and eating disorders are often a way they attempt to gain control over what they think they have little hold of. Eating disorders are not always about looks, which is what makes them so complex to shake off.

There is a difference between the two main eating disorders. Anorexia Nervosa is defined as a psychological illness characterized by self-image distortion and unhealthily low body weight. The disorder is also marked by a deep fear of gaining weight, which results in a person starving themselves and could also lead to an obsession with exercise. On the other hand, Bulimia Nervosa is more of a psychiatric condition where the patient binge eats (quickly eating unusually large amounts of food). It is then followed by remorse and guilt and the sufferer attempts to compensate for the binge by vomiting the food out, over-exercising or using diuretics, laxatives or enemas to purge the food eaten.

While treatment for eating disorders includes therapy and nutrition, among other key approaches, it is very important that the parents don't blame themselves. These problems can be very complex and not just due to one or two things like peer pressure or home environment, so it is not always likely that any parent would have a strong role to play.

In the general scheme of things, where physical appearances are concerned, boys are encouraged to look bigger whereas girls

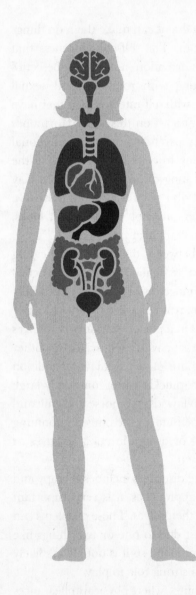

BRAIN
Symptoms include obsession with calorie counting, perpetual anxiety about gaining weight, fainting spells, headaches, mood swings, depression and dizziness.

SKIN and HAIR
Watch out for brittle nails, dry skin, dry lips, thinning hair, yellowish complexion, tendency to bruise easily, inability to withstand the cold, and thin white hair growth all over the body.

HEART
Anorexia could also show itself in irregular heart beat, low BP, heart failure/attacks and even poor circulation.

BLOOD
Anaemia (low levels of iron).

INTESTINES
Symptoms include bloating, diarrhoea, abdominal cramps and constipation.

HORMONES
Signs include problems with fertility and libido, as well as irregular periods.

KIDNEYS
Renal failure, dehydration.

BONES
Osteoporosis, osteopenia (bone calcium loss).

MUSCLES
Weakness, muscle loss, fatigue.

Signs and Symptoms of Anorexia Nervosa

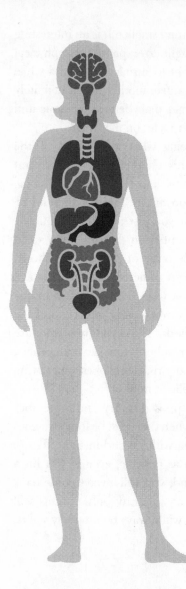

BRAIN
Symptoms include obsession with food and weight, perpetual anxiety, self-esteem issues and depression.

MOUTH
Bad breath, decay of teeth and enamel, gum problems, swollen jaws.

THROAT/OESOPHAGUS
Acid reflux/heartburn, inflammation/rupture of oesophagus, chronically sore throat.

HEART
Bulimia could also show itself in irregular heart beat, heart failure/attacks, low BP, dizziness and fainting spells.

INTESTINES
Symptoms include bowel issues, diarrhoea, abdominal cramps and constipation.

HORMONES
Signs include problems with fertility and libido, as well as irregular periods.

STOMACH
Stomach cramps, ulcers and, possibly, stomach rupture.

KIDNEYS
Dehydration.

SKIN
Dry skin, calluses (especially on the knuckles).

MUSCLES
Fatigue/tiredness, lethargy, cramps due to electrolyte imbalance.

Signs and Symptoms of Bulimia Nervosa

are encouraged to look thinner and smaller. It is an interesting observation that men are taught to expand their physical imprint while women are taught to shrink theirs. And while this is a conversation best continued another day, it definitely makes you think about the larger male–female dynamic and what this could mean for gender issues on the whole.

A child's growth curve being what it is, much of the information and advice in this chapter may be relevant earlier or later, depending on how your child is moving along. You may find this chapter more useful towards the end of your child's fourteenth year or you just might find yourself nodding vigorously in agreement from the time your child hits the tender age of ten. The onset of puberty has shown a shift and girls especially begin puberty at a younger age than previous generations. As a way to explain this unique phenomenon, there is a link between early puberty and the consumption of processed foods. Also, children who are overweight or obese may enter puberty quicker than others, but this is different for boys and girls. Being obese may bring forward puberty in girls but delay it in boys.[7]

As life moves on, as it is supposed to, try and remember what you were like at this age when there can be long stretches of perpetual misunderstanding with no end in sight. Try to dial in to your child as much as possible, even if you hit a few wrong numbers. In the end, you will always come back to loving your children with an intensity only parents will understand because your kids will always be uniquely yours, now and forever.

THE ABCs OF TEEN AND PRE-TEEN NUTRITION: TEN TO FIFTEEN YEARS

Chapter Summary

Nutritional guidance at this point is easy to give but hard to implement. You are not just dealing with peer influences, but your parenting has come head-to-head with a surge of hormones.

Puberty is your child's last big growth spurt and needs adequate nutrition to support it. The calorie requirements could extend upwards of 2000 from the age of ten onwards, which is more than some adults.

More calcium, zinc, protein, vitamins and better fats are needed to support this spurt of growth.

Nutrition needs to change for the Three As of an adolescent's life: athletics, academics and attitude. For the latter, you will be surprised at how foods can cause a shift in mood.

Eating disorders like Anorexia Nervosa and Bulimia Nervosa can start during the tender teen ages. While it is not that prevalent, do keep a lookout for the signs anyway.

Obesity can hasten the onset of puberty in girls and delay it in boys.

Rapunzel

A Tale of Nutritional Overprotection

In the fairy tale that is Rapunzel, which interestingly enough has no fairies, an evil witch locks up little Rapunzel in a high tower. With no way of getting in or out except for a window, the witch would reach her via climbing a rope made up of Rapunzel's long hair, resulting in the best shampoo advertisement that ever existed. While the moral of this story is that if you are light enough, you can climb hair, there exists a second moral: exercising too much control is pointless. In the end Rapunzel, all grown up and tired of being hemmed in, caught the fancy of a prince brave enough to set her free, and after a few plot twists, they lived happily ever after.

Sometimes locked away in towers are children who are living by too many rules and many of these include nutritional ones. 'Don't eat this', 'That is bad for you', 'This is so dirty', 'That has too many calories'. Nutritionist or not, I know my child shouldn't be eating a cupcake at a birthday party because of its near absence of any health benefit, but as I mentioned, in the ages six to nine chapter, once peer influence sets in, nutritional supervision can be done more successfully with a looser fist than an iron one.

But try telling that to many of the parents I meet. I have had both clients and friends who obsess over what their children eat in other people's houses, or put an embargo on whether they can eat with their friends. They travel abroad with ingredients like haldi, amchur, etc., and even take rice cookers and other cooking implements that suit the home cuisine better so that their children can eat healthy. To these parents, every dal is organic, every egg is free range and every roti has been made from happy organic grain harvested by happy farmers.

And yet, it is the same parents who can sometimes be the unhappiest.

Yes, I am with them on the free-range eggs and yes, the danger of processed ingredients cannot be emphasized enough. But the practice of eating right should never teeter on the brink of creating an inhospitable environment for food. Or compounding the stress in your own life. When it comes to teaching children about nutrition, associations with food should – as much as possible – not be negative ones. The more negative the association with food, the more complicated a relationship the child develops with it. And the longer a relationship, the more it perpetuates. Difficult relationships with food could translate into overeating, bingeing, starving and emotional eating, all of which is different from what the parent had originally intended.

While most would never sanction the addition of unhealthy foods in a child's diet, sometimes these items do slip in and sometimes even right under their noses. You can only control the eating environment when your children are in your sight, not when they aren't. Try as much to stick to the plan when you are out with them, and train them to make better choices when you are not. Don't work yourself up if they hit a few bumps along the road. Like Rapunzel, let down your hair, even if it is just a little bit, to prevent them from escaping the ivory tower and foregoing good nutritional habits altogether.

The End

Little Jack Horner

Childhood Obesity and What to Do About It

Kaveer was unlike any child I had ever met. A child of nine years brought in by his mother who was worried about his weight, he was bright, funny and wise way beyond his years. But only when someone took the time to sit him down and help him open up. Eleven kilos overweight on an otherwise slight frame, he had retreated into a shell that seemed to affect him both psychologically and academically. Like little Jack Horner, he sat in the corner during school recess, hoping to be spared the bullying for just one day, if he was lucky.

I am a nutritionist and not a psychologist, so I am only qualified to elaborate on the health aspects of weight gain, even though the psychological effects can stay with an overweight or obese child well after the weight has been shed. What I can tell you is that childhood obesity is globally on the rise, including in India. Look no further than the *Indian Journal of Endocrinology and Metabolism*, which states that anywhere between 5.74 per cent to 8.82 per cent of schoolchildren in India are obese.[1] The same report states that in urban South India, 21.4 per cent boys and 18.5 per cent girls who were aged thirteen to eighteen years were either overweight or obese.[2] There is also data here that says globally, the International Obesity Task Force (IOTF) has reported that in the year 2000, about 10 per cent of children aged five to seventeen years (so that is about 155 million) were overweight, out of which 2–3 per cent (about 30 to 45 million) were obese.[3] Additionally, another report states that 22 million children under five are obese.[4] Not overweight, but obese.

Of course, there are many reasons for obesity and you don't need to be a nutritionist to figure that out. The lack of exercise and an abundance of unhealthy cheaper foods are a few reasons. Or various social and environmental factors that affect both eating and physical activity, often called 'obesogenic' environments, could be others. Or maybe a genetic predisposition to gain weight. Whatever the reason for it, the ubiquity of unhealthy processed foods probably doesn't help and has led me, even as a nutritionist, to find a more moderate approach to supervising unhealthy foods which my children eat rather than banning them altogether. Despite what I believe. Despite what I want.

If your child is overweight or obese, the first thing you must do is not to let it affect your relationship with him. I have seen so many children come in with their parents, resentful of their efforts to make them lose weight, where the tension was so thick you could actually see it. Accusing your child of being lazy or ineffectual at losing weight is only going to put him on the defensive. Despite popular perception, restricting calorie intake is *not* the prescribed way to treat overweight young children.[5] Weight management at this young age is to arrest any further weight gain and also watch for growth in height with a view that overweight young children can grow into their height.

Overweight young children can grow into their height. The focus of managing obesity in younger age groups is more on *arresting weight gain* than losing weight.

However, yes, for those who have attained their height or are deemed close to the same as per their paediatrician, a healthy weight-loss diet and exercise are the only proven ways to lose the weight and keep it off. It is important to keep track of it and catch it early. An unbelievable 80 per cent of ten to fourteen-year-olds who are overweight are at a greater risk of struggling with weight gain as adults, as compared to only 25 per cent of overweight children under the age of five and 50 per cent of children aged six to nine.[6]

I just wanted to leave you with a final thought. Weight gain, despite a common misconception, is not necessarily caused by children who eat mountains of French fries at a time or have a milkshake marathon for a snack. Weight gain can occur in the smallest, most insidious ways, leading to the numbers gently creeping up on the scale. People who gain weight don't have to significantly overeat every day: even a little over the required norm can constitute excess consumption. Colas with dinner, chocolates for dessert, frequent eating of fast food could just, ever-so-slightly, tip the scales. It takes 3500 unburnt calories to gain a pound of weight. Even 100 extra calories (a cola or a few pieces of chocolate) per day that the child has not been able to burn could lead to 36,500 extra unburnt calories consumed per year, which is a weight gain of about 10 pounds or about 4 to 5 kilos. It is that frighteningly easy to gain weight. Whatever you do, find a way to negotiate this very tricky path with your child. It is a period that will need maximum sensitivity and effort.

The End

Feed This, Less That
Eating Out for Children

When it comes to eating out with your kid, you can't help but be assailed by numerous food choices wherever you may go, and not all of them are good. To prevent tantrums which would otherwise compel you to leave the venue covering your face with a napkin, I thought I could find you a way to balance the plate so that everybody wins. Needless to say, these foods may be contraindicated for some children with allergies and intolerances, so please go by the advice of your paediatrician.

As a revision of the 'Eating Out' guide in *Eat Delete*, the 'Feed This, Less That' guide in *Eat Delete Junior* has been tweaked for children and the adults who order food for them.

Birthday Parties

Feed This

- ☺ Idlis
- ☺ Live dosa counters
- ☺ Sandwiches – cheese/coleslaw/chicken
- ☺ Mini pizzas
- ☺ Noodles
- ☺ Pasta

Less That

- ☹ Candyfloss
- ☹ Carbonated beverages
- ☹ Cakes/cupcakes
- ☹ Chocolate-dipped/fondue marshmallows and candies
- ☹ Macaroons
- ☹ Chocolates and candies
- ☹ Cookies
- ☹ Jelly
- ☹ Ice creams
- ☹ French fries

Weddings and 'Grown-Up' Parties

Feed This

- ☺ Rice and dal
- ☺ Tandoori roti with vegetables

- ☺ Rice with curd/raita
- ☺ Noodles with vegetables or chicken
- ☺ Pasta
- ☺ Thai curry with rice
- ☺ Stuffed kulchas with dal or yogurt
- ☺ Tandoori chicken or paneer

Less That

- ☹ Falooda
- ☹ Kulfi
- ☹ Cakes and pastries
- ☹ Jalebis and gulab jamuns
- ☹ Fried samosas and pakoras
- ☹ Foods containing Ajinomoto/MSG. You may have to ask the host if MSG has been added to the food
- ☹ Foods which contain too much added food colour. Again, you may need to ask the host if the food contains food colour
- ☹ Pre-cut fruits and salads. When fruit is cut and left exposed to air, it gets oxidized and loses its nutritive value. Also, raw foods at room temperature spoil faster and may cause gastrointestinal discomfort

Restaurant Guide
Italian

Feed This

- ☺ Chicken or fish – either grilled, baked or broiled with lemon sauce on the side
- ☺ Pasta is one of the best ways to sneakily incorporate vegetables and any pasta like penne, spaghetti

or linguini in tomato or marinara sauce will be appropriate for your children. To get the best nutritional results out of it, ensure that the pasta dish has an equal proportion of pasta and vegetables. You can also add chicken, fish or turkey if your child likes it

☺ Clay-oven pizzas work well too. Not only do they give your child what they like, they also help you incorporate all the vegetables you want. You can order the pizza with tomato sauce and your choice of vegetables, chicken, seafood (above age two), fish (above age one), or turkey

Less That

☹ Fettuccine alfredo/bolognese. Alfredo is heavy in cream/cheese/white sauce while bolognese is a heavy meat-filled red sauce

☹ Lasagna/ravioli/cannelloni are high in fat, which is not surprising because they use cream and cheese

☹ Eggplant or chicken parmigiana. Parmigiana is pretty much the same as parmesan so again, it will be – like some of the jokes in this book – a bit too cheesy

☹ Fried calamari

☹ Gelato

☹ Tiramisu. It is rich in liqueur and mascarpone cheese

Chinese

Feed This

☺ Chicken/prawn/vegetable sui mai

☺ Seafood or vegetable cheung fun

☺ Prawn/chicken/vegetable dim sum

☺ Steamed bread or mushroom/chicken bun
☺ Wonton soup
☺ Chicken/vegetable noodle soup
☺ Steamed rice
☺ Fried rice
☺ American chopsuey
☺ Soft stewed rice with vegetables
☺ Soft stewed noodles
☺ Steamed prawns in lemon sauce
☺ Steamed fish in soya, ginger and spring onions
☺ Chicken/prawn/exotic vegetables in hunan sauce or oyster sauce. However, do ask the chef to ensure the vegetables, chicken or fish are boiled, sautéed and not fried

Less That

☹ Fried wontons
☹ Pork buns
☹ Salt-and-pepper fried chilly prawns
☹ Fried chilly chicken
☹ Sesame prawn toast
☹ Szechwan chicken
☹ Chicken/fish/vegetable manchurian
☹ Kung pao chicken/potato
☹ Chow mein and lo mein
☹ Golden fried prawns (anything with the word 'golden' in it is fried)
☹ 'Crispy' spinach chicken
☹ Black bean chicken
☹ Spring rolls
☹ Butter garlic prawns/chicken/vegetables

Thai

Feed This

- ☺ Chicken or fish satay with peanut sauce on the side
- ☺ Grilled chicken in Thai seasoning
- ☺ Pad Thai noodles
- ☺ Pad see ew
- ☺ Thai coconut soup
- ☺ Tom kha kai
- ☺ Panang chicken
- ☺ Kao pad (Thai fried rice)

Less That

- ☹ Spring rolls
- ☹ Curry puffs
- ☹ Moneybags
- ☹ Mee krob (crisp fried noodles)
- ☹ Sweet coconut rice
- ☹ Pla mouk tad (fried calamari)

Mexican

Feed This

- ☺ Burritos with black bean or pinto bean (not refried beans, please) with loads of vegetables and a dash of guacamole. It is another sneaky way to add vegetables to your child's meal
- ☺ Chicken or vegetable fajitas
- ☺ Quesadillas
- ☺ Gazpacho
- ☺ Enchiladas

Less That

- ☹ Nachos
- ☹ Flautas or taquitos. These soft tortilla wraps are loaded with meat and deep fried
- ☹ Chorizo
- ☹ Crunchy tacos

North Indian

Feed This

- ☺ Tandoori roti or naan (no butter)
- ☺ Roomali roti
- ☺ Plain/stuffed paratha, roti
- ☺ Pulao, biryani
- ☺ Palak paneer
- ☺ Steamed rice
- ☺ Yellow dal, but ask for less tadka
- ☺ Tandoori or grilled mushroom/baby corn/cauliflower/ paneer. Request for no basting with butter on top
- ☺ Tandoori chicken/fish/prawn tikka. Request for no basting after being removed from the tandoor
- ☺ Green salad, kachumber or raita
- ☺ Masala chaas
- ☺ Roasted papad
- ☺ Green chutney or water-based pickle

Less That

- ☹ Samosa and pakora
- ☹ Butter chicken/paneer
- ☹ Malai kofta, methi mattar malai
- ☹ Fried masala papad
- ☹ Oily aachar and sweet chutney

☹ Chicken or vegetable jalfrezi/achari
☹ Fish koliwada or any fried fish
☹ Dal makhani, dal fry

South Indian

Feed This

☺ Idli, idiyappam
☺ Sambhar
☺ Rava idlis
☺ Sada dosa, rava dosa, neer dosa, lapsi dosa, ragi dosa or Mysore masala dosa
☺ Tomato uttapam
☺ Appam
☺ Curd rice, lemon rice or tamarind rice
☺ Rawa upma
☺ Cabbage poriyal
☺ Avial
☺ Pongal

Less That

☹ Ghee idli, Kanchipuram idli, fried idli or Chettinad idli
☹ Medu vada, dahi vada, dal vada, sambhar vada, rasam vada
☹ Puri korma/bhaji
☹ Sandwich uttappam with cheese
☹ Sheera

Vacation/Holiday Eating

Feed This

- ☺ Low-fat milk
- ☺ Water
- ☺ White meat/turkey sandwiches with vegetables
- ☺ Small hamburger with vegetables (another great way to sneak these in)
- ☺ Broiled or grilled chicken sandwich
- ☺ Baked potatoes
- ☺ Pizza with vegetable toppings or cheese or both
- ☺ Fruits and vegetables
- ☺ Low-fat frozen yogurt (or fro-yo as the cool kids call it)
- ☺ Low-fat or fat-free salad dressings

Less That

- ☹ Colas, carbonated beverages and fruit drinks
- ☹ Sausages, pepperoni and hot dogs
- ☹ Anything fried, if possible, like fried chicken, chicken nuggets, potatoes or French fries
- ☹ Onion rings
- ☹ Bacon
- ☹ Salads with mayonnaise
- ☹ High-fat salad dressings like Thousand Island
- ☹ High-fat excess sugar foods

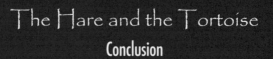

The Hare and the Tortoise
Conclusion

In *The Hare and the Tortoise*, the complacent hare, so confident that he could beat the slow tortoise in a clearly unfairly matched race, decided to nap right in the middle of said race – evidently someone's coach was also asleep at the wheel – only to wake up and find that the tortoise had beaten him to the punch. No matter how fast he ran, he couldn't win the race. He huffed and he puffed but he could not blow the house down.

Mixed metaphors aside, 'The Hare and the Tortoise', the concluding part to *Eat Delete Junior*, attempts to focus on the two main participants of the race: the hare and the tortoise. Every human being comes into this world with their unique bio-individuality and their own pace of development. Some babies blitz on so quickly that you can set your watch to the accuracy with which they reach their milestones. Others prefer to meander through life with the ease of a stroll in a garden, eventually reaching their destination in the end. Your child could be a hare, blazing a path of her own, or could be someone who prefers to stop and smell the roses. They are who they are, sometimes irrespective of who you would like them to be. And that is what makes them unique.

The overwhelming discourse – both implicit and explicit – about raising successful children seems to be associated with the achievement of goals, whether it is developmental, academic, social or eventually financial. First place, first car, first house. In this battle of always attempting to come first, it is also sometimes conveyed – again implicitly and explicitly – that being second, or third or last is not good enough. I do not agree with this idea. While nutrition is a vital partner in the development of a child's abilities, which in turn is a stepping stone to the achievement of his successes, I would like to leave you with one last concept: the difference between happiness and success.

I understand that most parents know this. I also understand that no matter what a child is taught about the concept of success, it is important to be happy; most parents would strive for their child's happiness above all else. Indeed, it was argued that success makes us happy, but we now know better than that. Ingrid Bergman famously and beautifully said that 'Success is getting what you want; happiness is wanting what you get.' To be successful at being happy requires us to better understand the idea of happiness. I thought I would take this idea further and establish the difference between happiness and success that I have observed over the years so that, like the nutritional advice in *Eat Delete Junior*, this may be one more thing parents could inculcate in their child, if they haven't already done so.

While nutrition will take your child places and can be influential in their success, happiness can be found no matter what is on your child's plate, wherever he or she may be. I have derived the most happiness from appreciating the tiniest moments with both my babies; whether it is remembering the time they spoke their first words or when their little hands made me a card for Mother's Day. With their happy, bouncy, limitless energy, younger children are especially brilliant at teaching us adults how to be happy. But as they grow older and realize the world can sometimes be a hard place to inhabit, they need to be reminded what they were so good at to begin with. Ultimately, like allowing them to judge their feelings of fullness as well as teaching them nutritional responsibility, how to be happy is something that I feel needs to be retaught on a regular basis so that your child is nourished, both inside and out.

Appendix

Recipes, Sample Diets and Food Presentation Ideas

I thought I would be tongue-in-cheek and put an actual picture of an appendix here since I have always found the usage of this vestigial organ in the context of the English language a little funny. Not sure why, though. However, it was easier said than done because finding one that didn't look so intimidating and science textbooky was, as it turns out, impossible. Ah, well.

This appendix is a treasure trove of recipes, meal ideas and meal plans, among other bits and bobs of useful information. As I have mentioned in the beginning of the book, do check in with your paediatrician, nutritionist or doctor before embarking on any nutritional programme. And wash all fruits and vegetables thoroughly to remove any traces of dirt before embarking on the preparation of the food.

The mini contents page rears its dashed head again here. Take a look:

I. Creating a Breast-Milk Bank[1]

Before handling or expressing breast milk, do the basics, like washing your hands with soap and water.

Storage

1. **Material:** To store expressed breast milk, you can choose either a glass container with a cap, a hard plastic BPA-free container or a special plastic bag designed for both the collection of milk and its storage. To those not in the know, BPA stands for Bisphenol A, an industrial chemical found in plastic containers that is known to leak and seep into foods or beverages. Exposure to BPA

has been linked to health and brain problems in foetuses, infants and children. Please don't store the breast milk in disposable bottle liners or any plastic bag made for general household use.

2. **Suitability:** To be honest, breast-milk storage bags may have a greater tendency to leak or tear than hard containers. But if you must use these storage bags, place them in a hard container with a working tight lid.

Method

1. Fill the breast milk in separate containers in quantities your baby will need for one feeding: about 60-120 ml. You could also store in smaller quantities (30-60 ml) for quicker feeds.

2. After you express the breast milk and transfer to your preferred container, put a label on it and write the date with a waterproof marker.

3. If you are storing it in the fridge, find a comfy place at the back because that is where the temperature is the coolest.

4. You can add freshly expressed milk to frozen or refrigerated milk so long as it has been expressed on the same day. Don't forget to cool the fresh milk in the fridge first before adding it to the previously chilled or frozen milk. Avoid adding warm breast milk to the frozen one because it may cause its colder cousin to partially thaw.

Life

How long breast milk keeps heavily depends on the method of storage.

1. At **room temperature**, fresh breast milk can be kept for up to six hours (four hours in a really warm room). But its use or storage within four hours is optimal.

2.   In an **insulated cooler** with ice packs, fresh milk can be stored for up to one day.

3.   In a **refrigerator,** fresh milk can be kept for up to five days in a clean space. However, its use or storage within three days is optimal.

4.   In a **deep freezer,** fresh milk can be stored **at the back** for up to a year. However, its usage within six months is optimal. Studies suggest, though, that the longer the breast milk is stored, the greater the loss of Vitamin C in the milk, so keep this mind. Also, do note that breast milk expressed when your child is a newborn will not be sufficient for a baby now a few months older. Guidelines for storage may also differ for pre-term, unwell or hospitalized babies.

Thawing

1.   Thaw the oldest batch first. You can do this by first transferring it to the fridge overnight so it gently changes state. Alternatively, the milk can be gently thawed by placing it in a bowl of warm water or simply under warm running water.

2.   Don't heat frozen breast milk in a microwave or on the stove. Studies suggest that quickly heating it can adversely affect the antibodies present in the milk. And while it is still not certain whether it is safe to refreeze previously frozen milk, many experts recommend that thawed milk be consumed within twenty-four hours.

3.   While thawed milk may smell slightly different or have a different consistency from fresh breast milk, it is still safe to give it to your baby. In case your baby refuses

to drink thawed breast milk, it may help to reduce the storage time.

II. Sample Lactation Diets (Breastfeeding)

These diets have been slightly modified from *Eat Delete*, with a view to making a balanced representation of nutrition. Every meal plan has been divided into main meals (breakfast, lunch, evening snack and dinner) with light 'fillers' in between. I prescribe eating every two hours, so the fillers can be used between main meals. Do note that 1 cup = 175 ml, 1 bowl = 180 ml and roti = 6 inch diameter.

1400 TO 1600 CALORIES

This is an approximation of a 1400 to 1600 calorie meal plan.
You would need to eat four main meals and four fillers.
Added oil (for cooking) should not exceed two to three teaspoons per day.

BREAKFAST

Choose any one option.

OPTION ONE:

- 1 bowl upma/poha with ½ bowl vegetables
- 1 glass vegetable juice
- 1 fruit

OPTION TWO:

- 1 vegetable sandwich
- ½ bowl cornflakes
- 1 cup skimmed milk
- 1 fruit

OPTION THREE:

- 2 slices bread
- 2 egg whites

- 1 glass vegetable juice
- 1 fruit

OPTION FOUR:

- 2 stuffed roti
- 1 bowl curd
- 1 fruit

LUNCH AND DINNER

Pick any two – one for lunch and one for dinner.

OPTION ONE:

- 3 roti
- 1 bowl dal OR ½ bowl dal and 1 cup curd
- 1 bowl vegetables

OPTION TWO:

- 2 roti
- ½ bowl steamed rice
- 1 bowl dal
- 1 bowl vegetables

OPTION THREE:

- 1 roti
- 1 bowl steamed rice
- 1 bowl dal
- ½ bowl curd
- 1 bowl vegetables

OPTION FOUR:

- 2 slices bread
- 1 bowl sprouts salad
- ½ bowl vegetable soup
- 2 vegetable cutlets

EVENING SNACK

Your evening snack should be a combination of any two filler items.

1600 TO 1800 CALORIES

This is an approximation of a 1600 to 1800 calorie meal plan.
You would need to eat four main meals and four fillers.
Added oil (oil for cooking) should not exceed two to four teaspoons per day.

BREAKFAST

Choose any one option.

OPTION ONE:

- 1 bowl upma/poha with ½ bowl vegetables
- 1 glass vegetable juice
- 1 fruit

OPTION TWO:

- ½ bowl cornflakes
- 1 vegetable sandwich
- 1 cup skimmed milk
- 1 fruit

OPTION THREE:

- 2 slices bread
- 2 egg whites
- 1 glass vegetable juice
- 1 fruit

OPTION FOUR:

- 2 stuffed roti
- 1 bowl curd
- 1 fruit

LUNCH AND DINNER

Pick any two – one for lunch and one for dinner.

OPTION ONE:

- 4 roti
- 1 bowl vegetables

- 1 bowl dal

OPTION TWO:

- 3 Roti
- ½ bowl steamed rice
- 1 bowl dal
- 1 bowl vegetables

OPTION THREE:

- 2 rotis
- 1 bowl steamed rice
- 1 bowl vegetables
- 1 bowl dal

OPTION FOUR:

- 2 slices bread
- 1 roti
- ½ bowl vegetable soup
- 1 bowl sprouts salad
- 2 vegetable cutlet

EVENING SNACK

Your evening snack should be a combination of any two filler items.

1800 TO 2000 CALORIES

This is an approximation of a 1800 to 2000 calorie meal plan.
You would need to eat four main meals and eight fillers.
Added oil (oil for cooking) should not exceed two to four teaspoons per day.

BREAKFAST

Choose any one option

OPTION ONE:

- 1 bowl upma/poha with ½ bowl vegetables
- 1 glass vegetable juice
- 1 fruit

OPTION TWO:

- ½ bowl cornflakes
- 1 vegetable sandwich
- 1 cup skimmed milk
- 1 fruit

OPTION THREE:

- 2 slices bread
- 2 egg whites
- 1 glass vegetable juice
- 1 fruit

OPTION FOUR:

- 2 stuffed roti
- 1 bowl curd
- 1 fruit

LUNCH AND DINNER

Pick any two — one for lunch and one for dinner.

OPTION ONE:

- 4 rotis
- 1 bowl vegetables
- 1 bowl dal

OPTION TWO:

- 3 rotis
- ½ bowl steamed rice
- 1 bowl vegetables
- 1 bowl dal

OPTION THREE:

- 2 rotis
- 1 bowl steamed rice
- 1 bowl vegetables

- 1 bowl dal

OPTION FOUR:

- 3 slices bread
- 1 roti
- ½ bowl vegetable soup
- 1 bowl sprouts salad
- 1 vegetable cutlet

EVENING SNACK

Your evening snack should be a combination of any two filler items.

2000 TO 2200 CALORIES

This is an approximation of a 2000 to 2200 calorie meal plan.
You would need to eat four main meals and eight fillers.
Added oil (oil for cooking) should not exceed two to four teaspoons per day.

BREAKFAST

Choose any one option

OPTION ONE:

- 2 bowl upma/poha with 1 bowl vegetables
- 1 glass vegetable juice
- 1 fruit

OPTION TWO:

- 1 bowl cornflakes
- 1 vegetable sandwich
- 1 cup skimmed milk
- 1 fruit

OPTION THREE:

- 3 slices bread
- 3 egg whites
- 1 glass vegetable juice
- 1 fruit

OPTION FOUR:

- 3 stuffed roti
- 1 bowl curd
- 1 fruit

LUNCH AND DINNER

Pick any two – one for lunch and one for dinner.

OPTION ONE:

- 4 rotis
- 1 bowl vegetables
- 1 ½ bowls dal

OPTION TWO:

- 3 rotis
- ½ bowl steamed rice
- 1 ½ bowls dal
- 1 bowl vegetables

OPTION THREE:

- 1 bowl steamed rice
- 2 rotis
- 1 bowl vegetables
- 1 ½ bowls dal

OPTION FOUR:

- 3 slices bread
- 1 roti
- ½ bowl vegetable soup
- 1 bowl sprouts salad
- 1 vegetable cutlet
- 1 cup curd

EVENING SNACK

Your evening snack should be a combination of any four filler items.

FILLERS

- 2 biscuits (Marie/KrackJack/Glucose/cream crackers/Monaco)
- 1 medium-sized diet khakra
- 1 medium-sized idli
- ½ medium sized sada dosa
- 17 grapes
- 6 to 8 strawberries
- 2 to 3 plums
- 18 to 20 cherries
- 4 medium slices of pineapple (diameter of the slice is approximately 3 inches)
- 1 medium-sized orange/apple/pear
- 6 to 7 lychees
- 1 bowl watermelon/muskmelon/papaya
- 1 bowl skimmed-milk curd
- 1 bowl kurmura (puffed rice)
- ½ bowl of sprouts salad
- Small fistful of channa and 1 glass chhaas
- 2 boiled egg whites and 1 cracker
- Vegetable juice
- ½ bowl of vegetable poha
- Open sandwich with vegetable toppings
- Chicken and peppers on bread
- ½ bowl of upma with beans and carrots
- ½ bowl of roasted poha chivda with some chana
- 2 tablespoons of cornflakes with skimmed milk
- ½ bowl of hakka noodles with veggies
- ½ bowl of pasta in red sauce with mushrooms
- ½ bowl of spaghetti with spinach
- 1 bowl of popcorn without butter
- Cornflakes bhel (2 tablespoons of corn/wheat flakes + 2 tablespoons of chopped vegetables)
- 1 tablespoon of hummus and 1 cracker

III. Introduction to Solids (Recipes)

How to Make Baby Rice/Dal Cereal from Scratch

I thought this was an exciting recipe which could be received well by your baby until the age of two years even. You could switch to a grainier texture when your baby reaches eighteen months of age.

Making the Cereal

Time Taken: Sixty to Ninety Minutes

- Step 1 | **Soak or Rinse**: Wash brown rice or white rice and dal separately until the water runs clear. Separately soak each in lots of water – uncovered in an airy place – for about six hours. Soaking rice and dal helps to break down their harder-to-digest components and also helps prevent an attack of colic. While soaking is better, if you are short on time, you can skip this step and go straight to just rinsing the rice and dal. Using a colander, drain each ingredient separately.

- Step 2 | **Air Dry**: Post draining, spread each ingredient out on a clean cloth, which is preferably white or undyed. Leave it to air dry or dry under a fan for thirty to fifty minutes.

- Step 3 | **Dry Roast**: On a medium flame, dry roast each ingredient separately for five minutes and then switch to a low flame till the rice or dal begins to pop and splutter. Then switch the stove off. Roasting helps make the cereal or grain gentler on the stomach. Wait for it to cool.

- Step 4 | **Powder and Store:** When cool, blend each to a fine powder. Keep the rice and dal separate. Store in an airtight jar.

Cooking the Cereal

Time Taken: Two Minutes

To prepare the cereal or any kind of baby food, always use a heavy-bottomed steel pot because the food needs to be cooked slowly so as to release the best texture and taste, and also to prevent burning. Mix one tablespoon of the above flour with ½ cup of water at room temperature; cook on a low flame, stirring constantly. A ratio of about one-part flour to six-parts water helps bring it to the right consistency, which should be just about right for your baby to consume. You may add more water to achieve this, if you like. When the cereal cools down, add formula milk or breast milk to enhance the nutrition, but just enough to maintain the desired consistency. If you are making a dal cereal, don't add milk; add ghee instead.

Stews

Stewed Apple

- Step 1 | Wash the apple thoroughly. Peel and cut into small bits.
- Step 2 | Put the chopped apple in a pan and add enough water to ensure the apple is fully submerged. Cook till soft.
- Step 3 | Once soft, remove from the pan and mash with a fork to get a smooth consistency.

Stewed Pear

- Same as stewed apple.

Stewed Carrot

- Step 1 | Peel and chop a small carrot into little pieces.
- Step 2 | Dunk the pieces in an open pan with enough water to cook the carrots till they are soft.
- Step 3 | Remove from the pan and put in a blender. Blend till smooth.
- Step 4 | Add a little unsalted butter for flavour.

Stewed Beetroot

- Same as stewed carrot.

Mashes

Mashed Banana

- Step 1 | Peel a ripe banana and cut into small pieces.

■ Step 2 | Mash with a fork.

■ Step 3 | Put the mashed bits in a blender and blend till smooth.

Mashed Chickoo

■ Step 1 | Peel and cut a ripe chickoo into small pieces. Discard the pip.

■ Step 2 | Puree the chickoo in a blender till smooth.

Mashed Papaya

■ Step 1 | Blend a few bits of chopped ripe papaya in a blender till you reach a smooth consistency.

Mashed Avocado

■ Step 1 | Scoop out the flesh of a ripe avocado. Discard the pip.

■ Step 2 | Blend till smooth.

■ Step 3 | You can add breast milk or formula to make it creamier.

Mashed Boiled Sweet Potato

■ Step 1 | Wash, peel and chop the sweet potato into big coarse pieces.

■ Step 2 | Dunk in a pressure cooker with water and cook for four to five whistles.

■ Step 3 | Remove from the cooker, mash and strain through a sieve to achieve a smooth consistency.

■ Step 4 | Add a little unsalted butter for flavour.

Other Recipes

Tomato and Pumpkin Soup

■ Step 1 | Chop one tomato and a piece of peeled pumpkin into small pieces. Put into a pressure cooker with water and cook for two to three whistles.

■ Step 2 | Remove from cooker and mash. Strain the contents through a sieve.

■ Step 3 | Add a little unsalted butter for flavour.

Rice Porridge

■ Step 1 | Mix one tablespoon of flour with 1/5 cup of water and cook over a low flame. Keep stirring to prevent the mixture from burning. You can add more water if needed.

■ Step 2 | When the cereal cools down, add breast milk or formula to enhance nutrition.

Ragi Porridge

■ Step 1 | In an open pan, heat a little ghee and roast the ragi flour (about half a teaspoon of ghee for two teaspoons of ragi). Keep stirring continuously till you get the aroma of it having roasted.

■ Step 2 | Take it off the heat and let it cool.

■ Step 3 | Now, add lukewarm water and mix well using a whisk. If water is added while the ragi is still hot, lumps will form.

■ Step 4 | Put it back on heat, whisking continuously till the mixture thickens.

■ Step 5 | Transfer from the pan to a bowl and add breast milk or formula for a thicker consistency.

Lentil Soup

■ Step 1 | Boil two tablespoons of moong dal in 1/5 cup of water with a pinch of turmeric until well cooked and soft. Mash the dal and add a 1/5 cup of water.

■ Step 2 | Boil again for a few minutes and strain the contents through a sieve to get a clear dal soup. Add a little unsalted butter for flavour.

Ragi Porridge with Bananas or Chickoo

■ Refer to the recipe for ragi porridge and add mashed banana or chickoo to it.

Sprouts and Vegetable Soup with Soft Boiled Rice Mash

■ Step 1 | Add sprouted moong to a mixture of vegetables like carrots, beans and potatoes.

■ Step 2 | Transfer the mix to a pressure cooker, add water and cook for approximately two whistles.

■ Step 3 | Cool and blend till it reaches a soup consistency.

■ Step 4| Add soft boiled and mashed rice.

■ Step 5 | A little bit of ghee or unsalted butter can be added for flavour.

Oats Porridge with Stewed Apples

- Step 1 | In an open pan, add 1/5 cup of organic oats and some water.
- Step 2 | After it comes to a boil, add oats and finely chopped pieces of apple. Allow it to cook.
- Step 3 | When fully done, remove from the flame and mash a little.

Vegetable Khichadi

- Step 1 | In a pressure cooker, heat ghee, add cumin seeds and let it splutter. Then add grated bottle gourd, grated carrot, moong dal and rice, followed by a pinch of turmeric.
- Step 2 | Sauté for a couple of minutes. Add just enough water and pressure cook for three whistles.
- Step 3 | Allow the steam to release. Mash the khichadi using the back of a spoon.

Spinach Moong Dal with Soft Boiled Rice Mash

- Step 1 | In an open pan, heat ghee, add cumin seeds and let it crackle. Add some moong dal, spinach, turmeric and water. Cook till it is well done.
- Step 2 | Mash well. Mix it with soft boiled and mashed rice.

Mixed Vegetable Rava Upma

- Step 1 | In an open pan, heat ghee. Add a few mustard seeds and three to four curry leaves. Let them crackle.
- Step 2 | Add semolina and roast for three to four minutes on medium flame. Add boiling water, which should be enough to achieve a runny consistency.
- Step 3 | Add one soft-boiled vegetable to this – carrots/beans/pumpkin/bottle gourd. Mix it well.

Idli with Mixed Vegetable Soup

- Step 1 | Make soft idlis with home-made batter.
- Step 2 | Refer to the vegetable soup recipe. Dunk the idlis in it.

Scrambled Egg Yolk with Soft Bread

- Step 1 | Separate the white from the egg yolk; discard the egg white. Beat the egg yolk till light and fluffy.

- Step 2 | Heat some butter in a pan, add the yolk and stir continuously on medium heat till cooked (the scramble should be soft, not overdone).
- Step 3 | Heap the cooked egg on a fresh slice of soft bread.

Aloo Paratha Dipped in Yogurt

- Step 1 | In a mixing bowl, add wheat flour, soft-boiled and mashed potato, finely chopped onion, finely chopped fresh coriander, ghee and water (if required).
- Step 2 | Knead it into a soft dough and roll out thick rotis.
- Step 3 | On a heated pan, roast the paratha on both sides till almost cooked. Apply ghee on both sides and fry for a minute more. Serve with fresh yogurt.

Vegetable Noodle Soup

- Step 1 | Add vegetables like carrots, beans, potato and bottle gourd to a pan.
- Step 2 | Add some water and simmer to make a clear vegetable stock.
- Step 3 | Strain the stock and discard the vegetables. Add boiled noodles to the stock and simmer for two minutes.

Paneer and Vegetable Paratha

- Step 1 | Make fresh paneer at home by curdling the milk.
- Step 2 | Mash the paneer and add finely chopped onion, chopped fresh coriander and any boiled vegetable like carrot/bottle gourd/grated pumpkin/potato to it. Mix it together.
- Step 3 | Make a soft dough with wheat flour.
- Step 4 | Roll out a roti, put the mixture in the centre of it, reshape and roll again.
- Step 5 | Roast it on a pan. Apply ghee to both sides and fry for a minute.

Avocado Mash with Buttered Bread

- Step 1 | Refer to the recipe for an avocado mash.
- Step 2 | On a fresh soft slice of bread, apply unsalted butter and top with avocado mash.

Soft Dosa/Uttapam or Steamed Idli with Dal

- Step 1 | With home-made batter, make any one: a soft dosa, uttapam or steamed idli.
- Step 2 | For the dal, heat a little ghee, add whole jeera, moong dal, a pinch of turmeric and enough water to cook the dal.
- Step 3 | Mash the dal well and serve with dosa/uttapam/idli.

Moong Dal Chillas with Yogurt

- Step 1 | To a tablespoon of moong dal flour, add chopped onions, a little fresh coriander, finely chopped tomatoes and enough water to make a pouring consistency.
- Step 2 | Heat a pan and spread the mixture out like a pancake. Apply ghee to both sides till cooked.
- Step 3 | Serve with fresh yogurt.

Oats and Vegetable Chilla

- Step 1 | Mix together the oats, grated and boiled carrot/bottle gourd/pumpkin/ sweet potato and finely chopped fresh coriander. Make a batter which has pouring consistency.
- Step 2 | Heat a pan and spread the mixture out like a pancake. Apply butter on either side till cooked.

Pasta with Boiled Vegetables

- Step 1 | In an open pan, heat unsalted butter. Add boiled pasta and a pinch of mixed herbs.
- Step 2 | Add steamed vegetables like carrots, beans, green peas and broccoli. Toss well for a minute and serve.

Curd Rice

- Step 1 | Cook rice until soft. Wait for it to cool.
- Step 2 | Beat fresh yogurt and temper it with mustard seeds and a few curry leaves. Add it to the cooled rice and mix well.
- Step 3 (Optional) | Steamed and grated carrot can also be added.

IV. Pre-teen and Teen Nutrition: Sample Diets for Ten to Fifteen-Year-Olds

Listed are some indicative meals plans for children aged ten to fifteen. I've divided these into meal plans for children aged ten to twelve years (because the calorie requirement difference between boys and girls at this age is minor) and separate diets for boys and girls aged thirteen to fifteen years. Do note that 1 cup = 175 ml, 1 bowl = 180 ml and roti = 6 inch diameter.

SAMPLE DIET FOR CHILDREN AGE TEN TO TWELVE
YEARS (2000–2200 CALORIES)

Oil: Two to four teaspoons
Four main meals + eight fillers

BREAKFAST OPTIONS

Choose any one.

OPTION ONE:

- 2 cup skimmed milk
- Granola – 3 heaped tablespoons
- 1 fruit

OPTION TWO:

- 2 toasts
- 1 tablespoon peanut butter on toast
- 1 fruit

OPTION THREE:

- 2 toast + 1 slice low fat cheese
- 2 egg white + 1 yolk
- 1 cup skimmed milk

OPTION FOUR:

- 3 stuffed rotis
- 1 bowl curd
- 1 fruit

OPTION FIVE:

- 2 bowls upma/poha with 1 bowl vegetables
- 1 glass veggie juice
- 1 fruit

LUNCH AND DINNER OPTIONS

Choose any one for dinner and one for lunch.

OPTION ONE:

- 4 rotis
- 1 bowl vegetables
- 1 ½ bowls dal

OPTION TWO:

- 2 rotis
- 1 bowl rice
- 1 bowl vegetables
- 1 ½ bowls dal

OPTION THREE:

- 1 bowl soup
- 1 bowl pasta with 1 bowl vegetables/salad
- Chicken (boneless 100g) or paneer (30g)
- 2 slices of (garlic or herb) bread

OPTION FOUR:

- 1 bowl soup
- 1 bowl noodles with 1 bowl vegetables
- 1 bowl rice sautéed with vegetables and 2 egg whites, scrambled
- Chicken (100g) or paneer(30g) in any Chinese sauce (less oil)

OPTION FIVE:

- 2 sandwiches with chicken slices (100g) or paneer (30g)
- 1 bowl soup
- 1 bowl salad

EVENING SNACK

Evening snack is combination of four fillers.
Please refer to the list of fillers on page 206.

SAMPLE DIET FOR GIRLS AGE THIRTEEN TO FIFTEEN YEARS (APPROXIMATELY 2200-2400 CALORIES)

Oil: two to four teaspoons
Four main meals + eight fillers

BREAKFAST

Choose any one option.

OPTION ONE:

- 1 bowl oatmeal with milk
- 15 raisins + 5 walnuts (halves) + 1 tablespoon honey
- 2 boiled eggs (1 yolk + 2 whites)
- 1 fruit

OPTION TWO:

- 3 eggs, scramble (1 yolk + 3 whites)
- 2 toasts + 1 slice low fat cheese
- 1 cup skimmed milk
- 1 fruit

OPTION THREE:

- 2 idlis
- 1 masala dosa
- 1 bowl sambhar
- 2 tablespoons coconut chutney

OPTION FOUR:

- 3 stuffed rotis
- 1 bowl curd
- 1 fruit
- 1 glass veggie juice

LUNCH AND DINNER

Choose any one for dinner and one for lunch.

OPTION ONE:

- 3 rotis
- 1 bowl steamed rice
- 1 bowl vegetables
- 1 ½ bowl dal
- 1 cup curd

OPTION TWO:

- 1 bowl soup
- 2 small burger breads with chicken (150g boneless) or potato + paneer (45g) fillet and vegetables
- 1 slice low fat cheese (half slice per burger)
- 1 bowl salad

OPTION THREE:

- 1 bowl soup
- 1 ½ bowls spaghetti with 1 bowl vegetables/salad
- Chicken (boneless 150g) or paneer (45g)
- 3 slices of (garlic or herb) bread

OPTION FOUR:

- 4 rotis
- 1 ½ bowl vegetable
- 1 ½ bowls dal
- 1 bowl curd

EVENING SNACK

Evening snack is combination of four fillers.
Please refer to the list of fillers on page 206.

SAMPLE DIET FOR BOYS AGE THIRTEEN TO FIFTEEN YEARS (APPROXIMATELY 2800 CALORIES)

Oil: two to four teaspoons
Four main meals + eight fillers

BREAKFAST

Choose any one option.

OPTION ONE:

- 1 ½ bowl oatmeal with milk
- 15 raisins + 5 walnuts (halves) + 1tbsp honey
- 3 boiled eggs (1 yolk + 3 whites)
- 1 fruit

OPTION TWO:

- 4 egg scramble (1 yolk + 4 whites)
- 3 toasts + 1 slice low fat cheese
- 1 cup skimmed milk
- 1 fruit

OPTION THREE:

- 4 idlis
- 1 masala dosa
- 1 bowl sambhar
- 2 tablespoons coconut chutney

OPTION FOUR:

- 3 stuffed roti
- 2 bowl curds
- 2 fruit
- 1 glass veggie juice

LUNCH AND DINNER IDEAS

Pick any one for lunch and one for dinner.

OPTION ONE:

- 4 rotis

- 1 bowl steamed rice
- 1 bowl vegetables
- 2 bowl dal
- 1 cup curd

OPTION TWO:

- 1 ½ bowl soup
- 2 small burger breads with chicken (200g boneless) or potato + paneer (60g) fillet and vegetables
- 1 slice low fat cheese (half slice per burger)
- 1 ½ bowl salad

OPTION THREE:

- 1 bowl soup
- 2 bowl spaghetti with 1 ½ bowl vegetables/salad
- Chicken (boneless 200g) or paneer (60g)
- 3 slices of (garlic or herb) bread

OPTION FOUR:

- 4 rotis
- 2 bowl vegetable
- 1 ½ bowls dal
- 2 bowl curds

EVENING SNACK

Evening snack is combination of four fillers.
Please refer to the list of fillers on page 206.

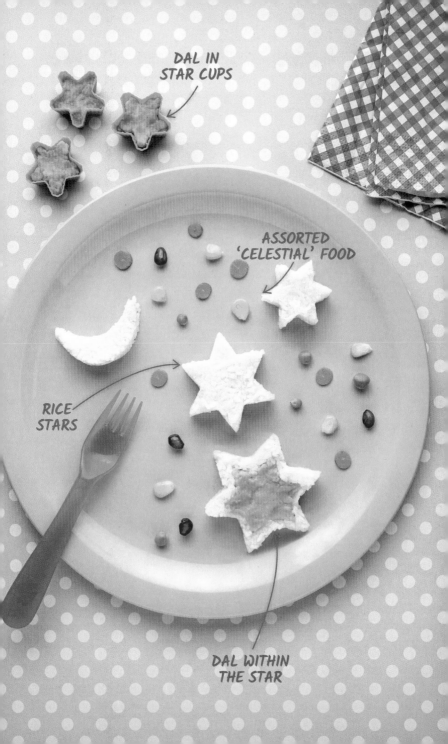

DAL IN
STAR CUPS

ASSORTED
'CELESTIAL' FOOD

RICE
STARS

DAL WITHIN
THE STAR

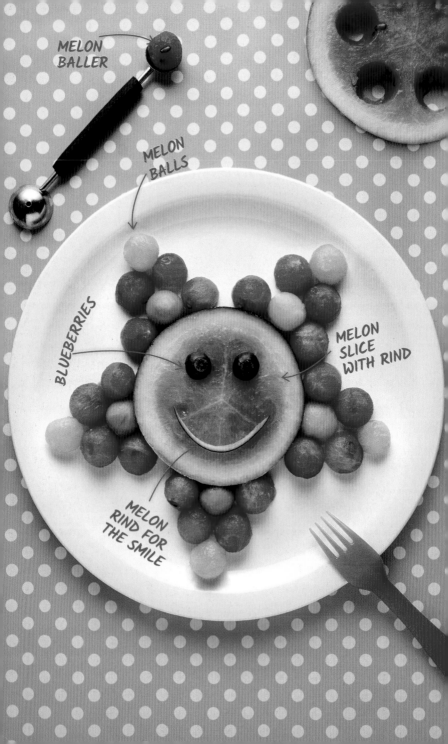

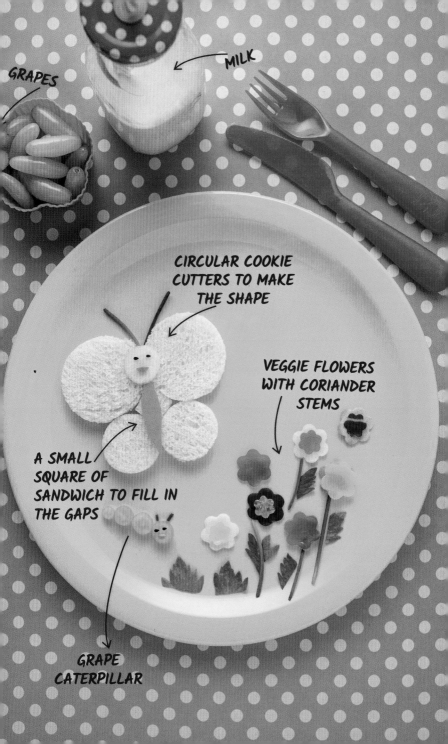

GRAPES

MILK

CIRCULAR COOKIE CUTTERS TO MAKE THE SHAPE

VEGGIE FLOWERS WITH CORIANDER STEMS

A SMALL SQUARE OF SANDWICH TO FILL IN THE GAPS

GRAPE CATERPILLAR

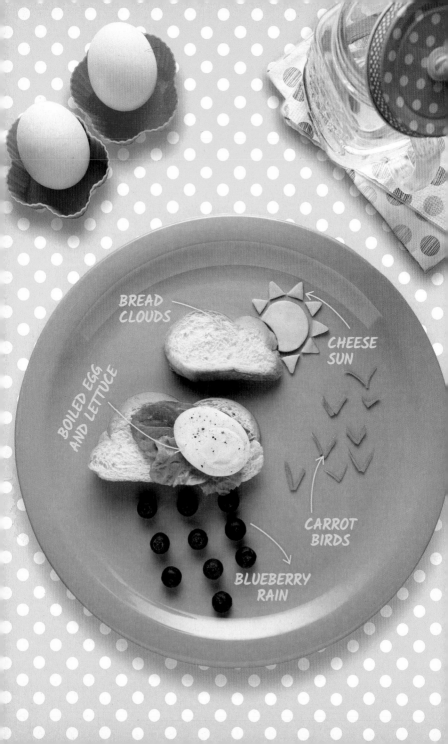

BREAD CLOUDS

CHEESE SUN

BOILED EGG AND LETTUCE

CARROT BIRDS

BLUEBERRY RAIN

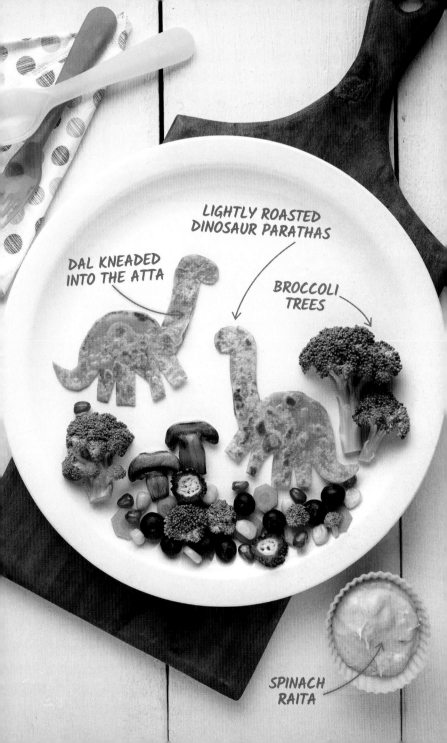

LIGHTLY ROASTED
DINOSAUR PARATHAS

DAL KNEADED
INTO THE ATTA

BROCCOLI
TREES

SPINACH
RAITA

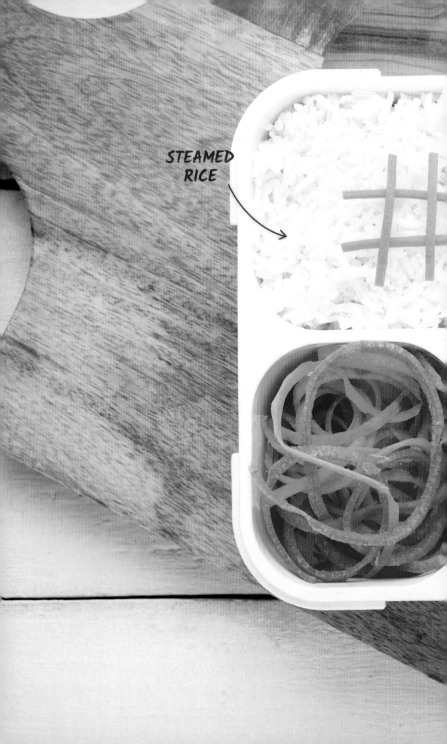

STEAMED
RICE

ou are what you eat!

HERBED
CHICKEN

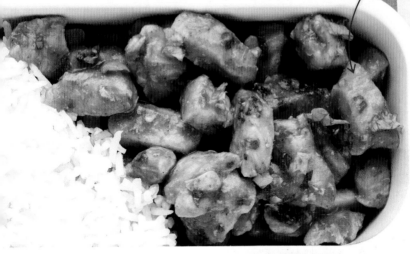

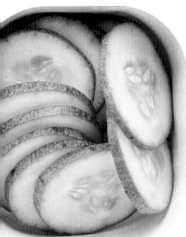

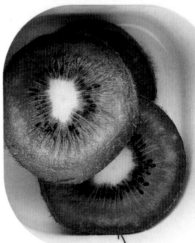

ASSORTED
FRESH VEGETABLES
AND FRUIT

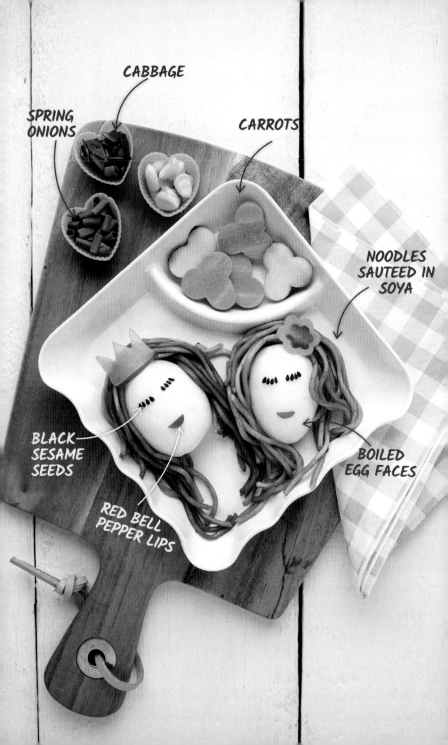

SPRING
ONIONS

CABBAGE

CARROTS

NOODLES
SAUTEED IN
SOYA

BLACK
SESAME
SEEDS

RED BELL
PEPPER LIPS

BOILED
EGG FACES

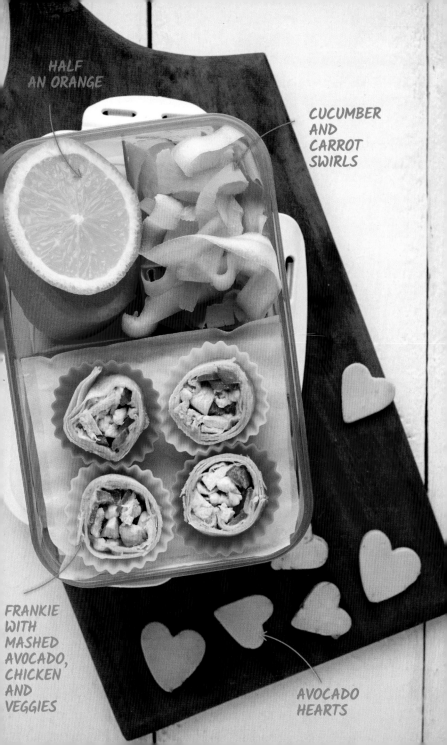

HALF
AN ORANGE

CUCUMBER
AND
CARROT
SWIRLS

FRANKIE
WITH
MASHED
AVOCADO,
CHICKEN
AND
VEGGIES

AVOCADO
HEARTS

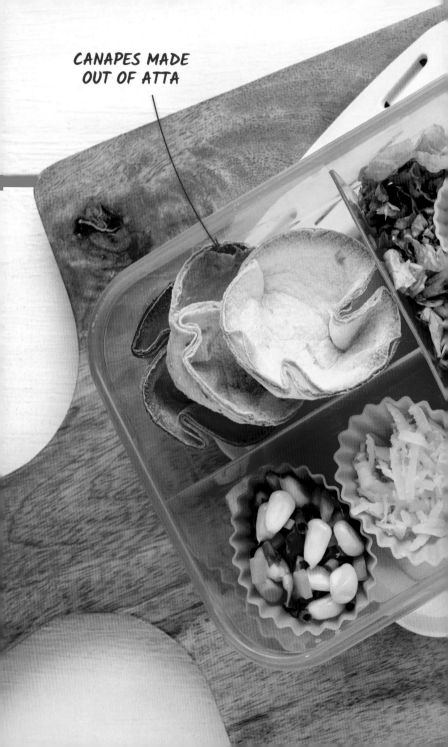

CANAPES MADE
OUT OF ATTA

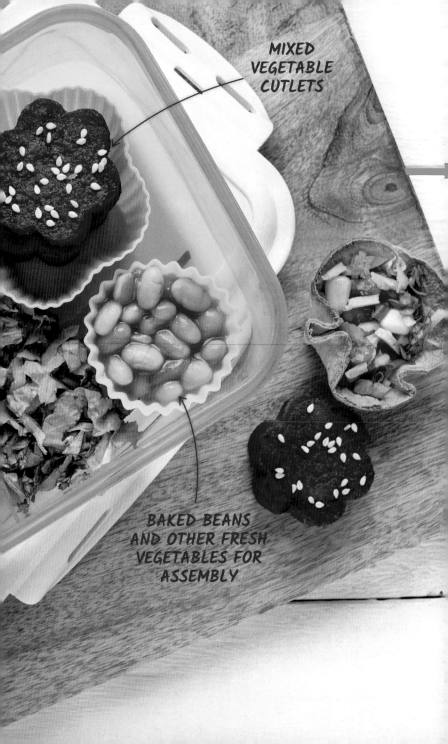

MIXED
VEGETABLE
CUTLETS

BAKED BEANS
AND OTHER FRESH
VEGETABLES FOR
ASSEMBLY

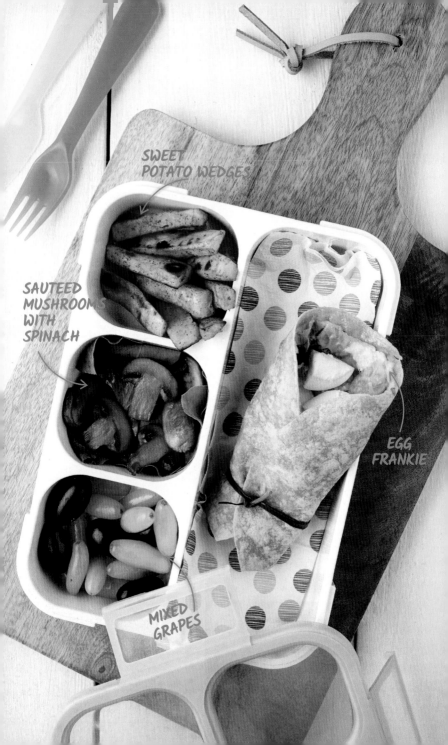

SWEET POTATO WEDGES

SAUTEED MUSHROOMS WITH SPINACH

EGG FRANKIE

MIXED GRAPES

End Notes

Alice in Wonderland

1. Called the Real Mothers Heard survey, directed by Baby Dove across five other countries to include the US, the UK, China, Brazil and Mexico.
2. http://timesofindia.indiatimes.com/city/mumbai/Dove-launches-baby-care-products/articleshow/54676816.cms; Last accessed on 19 April 2017.

3. http://food.ndtv.com/health/your-baby-requires-5-times-more-food-than-you-for-healthy-growth-1661357; Last accessed on 19 April 2017.

Breastfeeding

1. https://www.psychologytoday.com/blog/headshrinkers-guide-the-galaxy/201312/how-make-mountain-out-molehill.

2. https://www.healthychildren.org/English/ages-stages/baby/breastfeeding/Pages/Breastfeeding-After-Cesarean-Delivery.aspx; Last accessed on 19 April 2017.

3. Ibid.

4. http://www.infantnutritioncouncil.com/resources/breastmilk-information/; Last accessed on 19 April 2017.

5. Ibid.

6. Ibid.

7. http://news.health.com/2014/03/31/3-things-you-need-to-know-about-alcohol-and-breastfeeding; Last accessed on 19 April 2017.

8. https://www.psychologytoday.com/blog/prime-your-gray-cells/201109/the-skinny-brain-fats; Last accessed on 20 March 2017.

9. http://www.mhhe.com/biosci/ap/vander/student/olc/d-reading3.html; Last accessed on 19 April 2017.

10. Ibid.

11. Ibid.

12. https://www.ncbi.nlm.nih.gov/pmc/articles/PMC2812877/; Last accessed on 19 April 2017.

13. http://www.mayoclinic.org/healthy-lifestyle/infant-and-toddler-health/in-depth/breast-milk-storage/art-20046350?pg=2; Last accessed on 19 April 2017.

14. http://www.nhs.uk/conditions/pregnancy-and-baby/pages/types-of-infant-formula.aspx; Last accessed on 15 February 2017.

15. https://www.ncbi.nlm.nih.gov/pmc/articles/PMC2812877/; Last accessed on 19 April 2017.

Once Upon a Time

1. http://timesofindia.indiatimes.com/life-style/health-   fitness/ health-news/India-is-the-diabetes-capital-of-the-world/ articleshow/50753461.cms; Last accessed on 19 April 2017.

Introduction to Solids

1. https://www.ncbi.nlm.nih.gov/pubmed/19685855; Last accessed on 19 April 2017.
2. http://www.nhs.uk/Conditions/pregnancy-and-baby/Pages/ solid-foods-weaning.aspx; Last accessed on 19 April 2017.
3. http://wholesomebabyfood.momtastic.com/howmuchbabyeat. htm; Last accessed on 19 April 2017.
4. https://www.nhs.uk/start4life/first-foods; Last accessed on 21 February 2017.
5. https://www.nhs.uk/start4life/first-foods#recomms; Last accessed on 21 February 2017
6. https://medlineplus.gov/ency/article/007618.htm; last accessed on 21 February 2017.

Sleeping Beauty

1. https://sleepfoundation.org/sleep-topics/children-and-sleep; Last accessed on 19 April 2017.
2. https://www.ncbi.nlm.nih.gov/pubmed/11952652; Last accessed on 19 April 2017.

Early Childhood Nutrition

1. http://www.pubs.ext.vt.edu/content/dam/pubs_ext_vt_
   edu/348/348-150/348-150_pdf.pdf; Last accessed on 19 April
   2017.

The Little Mermaid

1. http://www.naturalhydrationcouncil.org.uk/wp-content/
   uploads/2013/09/Hydration-for-Children.pdf; Last accessed on
   19 April 2017.
2. Ibid.
3. http://www.who.int/water_sanitation_health/dwq/
   nutrientschap3.pdf; Last accessed on 19 April 2017.

The Princess and the Pea

1. Kelly Dorfman, What's Eating Your Child?: The Hidden
   Connections Between Food and Childhood Ailments, New York:
   Workman Publishing, 2011.
2. http://www.livestrong.com/article/539232-kids-symptoms-of-
   gluten-intolerance/; Last accessed on 19 April 2017.
3. http://kidshealth.org/en/parents/lactose.html; Last accessed on
   19 April 2017.
4. Kelly Dorfman, What's Eating Your Child?: The Hidden
   Connections Between Food and Childhood Ailments, New York:
   Workman Publishing, 2011.

Rip Van Winkle

1. http://icmr.nic.in/final/rda-2010.pdf; Last accessed on 19 April
   2017.
2. Ibid.

Hansel and Gretel

1. http://brandequity.economictimes.indiatimes.com/news/ advertising/82-children-are-influenced-by-product-ads-study/56057814; Last accessed on 19 April 2017.

2. http://www.independent.co.uk/environment/climate-change/ pester-power-the-new-weapon-in-the-fight-against-global-warming-10292998.html; Last accessed on 19 April 2017.

Pre-Teen and Teen Nutrition

1. https://www.ncbi.nlm.nih.gov/pmc/articles/PMC4266867/; Last accessed on 19 April 2017.

2. http://www.epi.umn.edu/let/pubs/img/adol_ch1.pdf; Last accessed on 19 April 2017.

3. http://pediatric-house-calls.djmed.net/puberty-tanner-stages-boys/; Last accessed on 19 April 2017.

4. https://www.ncbi.nlm.nih.gov/pmc/articles/PMC4266867/; Last accessed on 19 April 2017.

5. http://icmr.nic.in/final/RDA-2010.pdf; Last accessed on 19 April 2017.

6. https://childdevelopmentinfo.com/adhd-add/five-foods-negatively-affect-childs-mood/#.WGZgj7Z97aI; Last accessed on 19 April 2017.

7. https://www.ncbi.nlm.nih.gov/pubmed/24190685?report=abstract; Last accessed on 19 April 2017.

Little Jack Horner

1. https://www.ncbi.nlm.nih.gov/pmc/articles/PMC3063535/; Last accessed on 19 April 2017.

2. Ibid.

3. Ibid.

4. https://www.ncbi.nlm.nih.gov/pmc/articles/PMC4367021/; Last accessed on 19 April 2017.

5. https://www.ncbi.nlm.nih.gov/pmc/articles/PMC3063535/; Last accessed on 19 April 2017.

6. Ibid.

Appendix

1. http://www.mayoclinic.org/healthy-lifestyle/infant-and-toddler-health/in-depth/breast-milk-storage/art-20046350?pg=2; Last accessed on 19 April 2017.

Acknowledgements

It takes a village to raise a book. *Eat Delete Junior* would have been but an unrealized dream if it weren't for the help and good wishes of:

Ravi, my husband, best friend, life partner and support. I am who I am because of your belief in me.

Ahaana and **Amaira** – my badi and chotti – my two daughters, who inspired this book and who continue to inspire me every single day. I am so proud of the young women you are growing up to be.

My two pillars **Mom** and **Mumma**, who have given birth to a daughter-in-law and daughter respectively. Thank you for never failing to be present when I have been absent.

My **Dad** and **Pa**. Your guidance and advice have proved invaluable. Thank you so much for your strength.

My little brother **Aakash**. Thank you for unleashing the genie trapped within Nourish. Thank you for www.nourishgenie.com, one of the best gifts I have ever received.

My little sister **Ekta**, the bestest sister in the world. Thanks for giving me the gift of little Arjun, to whom I will always be B Mumma. And am so excited to meet the bun in the oven.

My paediatrician **Dr Ravinder Chittal**. Thank you for always being there for my girls, day or night. And for your contribution to this book.

My amazing **clients**, both grown-up and little. Thank you for making me the nutritionist I am today. I have learnt so much from you all. But just because you're fabulous doesn't mean you stop eating every two hours.

Debasri Rakshit, Commissioning Editor at HarperCollins. Thank you for being the fount of wisdom and enthusiasm that you are. And for laughing at all the jokes, good and bad.

Rea Mukherjee, Assistant Editor at HarperCollins. Thank you for your passion for the intricacies and hidden nuances of the English language. The book is so much better because of it.

Deepa Khatri, friend, partner-in-crime, graphic designer. Thank you so much for making *Eat Delete Junior*'s cover what it is.

Jojy Philip, typesetter.

Beynaz Mistry and Amrita Kaur, food photographer and food stylist respectively. You brought our recipes to life.

Dr Rakesh Sinha, doctor and inspiration. Thank you for not only making my journey to motherhood seamless but also for teaching me how to be a useful human being. May your beautiful soul rest in peace.

Team Nourish and **Team Nourish Genie**. You are indispensable, and I owe you a deep debt of gratitude.

My writer **Gayatri Pahlajani** for knowing me inside out. Thank you for being able to echo exactly what I am thinking even before I say it. For being my angel, my shadow and my light. No words can do justice for the gratitude I have for you.

To the many, many people I didn't name but whom I know I owe so much, thank you for your presence in my life. You've helped me more than you'll ever know.